Concussion Management for Primary Care

Deepak S. Patel
Editor

Concussion Management for Primary Care

Evidence-Based Answers to Cases
and Questions

Second Edition

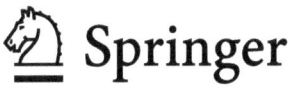 Springer

Editor
Deepak S. Patel
Family and Sports Medicine
Rush University Medical Center
Aurora, IL, USA

ISBN 978-3-031-85515-3   ISBN 978-3-031-85516-0   (eBook)
https://doi.org/10.1007/978-3-031-85516-0

This Springer imprint is published by the registered company Springer Nature Switzerland AG
The registered company address is: Gewerbestrasse 11, 6330 Cham, Switzerland

If disposing of this product, please recycle the paper.

Preface

Concussions are very common for providers in various practice settings. The high frequency of concussions may be fueled by increased media exposure and overall public and provider awareness. Regardless of the cause, medical providers are called upon to accurately diagnose and manage these concussions. Adding to this pressure is the fact that each state in the United States has some variation of legislation on management of concussions in children. These factors strengthen the need for primary care providers to be well-versed in the evaluation and management of them.

Although evidence in medicine changes and expands rapidly, this text aims to provide the latest update. The second edition includes updated evidence and advances in concussion care. Early guidelines were based on expert opinion. Interest in scientific research studies on concussions has provided better recommendations for providers. As this new evidence has become available, guidelines have been revised. This evidence has challenged several facets of concussion care and even refuted prior long-held beliefs. Despite this evidence, there are still areas of concussion care that long for better evidence and may be challenging to implement logistically.

This text provides primary care physicians and clinicians with an evidence-based yet practical approach to diagnosing and treating concussions in children and adults. Each of the authors were carefully selected based on their expertise and experience in managing concussions. In addition to being experts, they also serve as educators on concussions.

The book begins with a general overview of concussions. It then identifies concussions risks, signs, and symptoms. Next, physicians and providers learn when and how to perform appropriate physical exams for suspected concussions. The following chapters focus on selecting the correct type of testing to perform in suspected concussions. The testing options addressed include diagnostic, neurocognitive, and imaging. Return-to-learn and return-to-play recommendations are then discussed to ensure that providers are able to properly educate patients about the safe return. The book concludes by explaining post-concussion syndrome and identifying methods to prevent concussions and complications in the future.

Each chapter presents a specific real-world patient case and addresses common questions asked by patients and family. Within each chapter are additional follow-up questions in the subsections that help the reader to answer questions. Tables and a summary of key concepts have been included for readers looking for rapid specifics.

Presented from the unique perspective of primary care physicians who also specialize in sports medicine and concussions, *Concussion Management for Primary Care* is a first-of-its-kind book that serves as a valuable resource for primary care providers, sports medicine physicians, and any other clinician treating patients suffering from a possible concussion. Due to the success of the first edition, this second edition follows a similar format and incorporates updates on the latest evidence on concussion care.

Chicago, IL, USA   Deepak S. Patel
Aurora, IL, USA
Yorkville, IL, USA

Acknowledgments

This textbook is a culmination of effort and sacrifice from several individuals. I wanted to graciously acknowledge a few of the many involved.

Most important is the love, support, and sacrifices from my family (my wonderful wife and daughter). They are the reason I'm able to pursue an extensive project such as this. Their love and understanding helped me through this process. To my family I say, your understanding and support keeps me going every day, especially on a long commitment such as this. You push me to be my best and love me just the same when I'm not. Amazingly, you both have understood the importance of concussions and how my work might contribute to that. You were able to envision the benefit to others as you sacrificed and supported me in such a challenging project. Please know that there were many times when I was working on this project that I wished I was able to spend more time with you. I love you and am eternally grateful.

My next dedication is to my parents. Although both have passed, they are still always in my thoughts. I'm grateful for the person and especially the physician they helped me become. They taught me the value of hard work and persistence. They instilled the value of always learning and growing. Additionally, they helped me to love being a physician by caring for the sick and injured, but also to realize the importance of treating patients like family. This book is a reflection of those values.

Although I've taken on several different teaching roles, I am grateful for all of them. Whether I was teaching physicians colleagues, fellows, residents, medical students, nurse practitioners, physician assistants, nurses, athletic trainers, patients, or patients' family members, I appreciated that opportunity. Each of them has taught me something and pushed me to expand my knowledge. Along with their teachings, I want to thank all of them for their trust. Because of their trust, I've been privileged to demonstrate a vast array of experience in concussion care.

I want to thank each of the authors who have invested numerous hours of their personal time to lend their expertise to this work and help advance the state of education on concussions. Each of them is busy in their practice and teaching roles. I know this book was an extra responsibility that reduced their personal or family time. Thank you for your dedication and effort!

Each of us has unique experiences that shaped our interests and career choices. I had several of these, including sports injuries that pushed me toward a career in sports medicine. I firmly believe these can give us empathy for our patients. There is one experience specific to concussions that I wanted to share. In this and many regards, I wish to also thank my seventh and eighth-grade football coach and neighbor, Jerry Nichols. He probably was unaware of all the life lessons he taught his athletes and that a concussion to a future sports medicine physician would be one of them. During a practice, he chose to run a trick play, where the guard who was approximately a 6-foot, 200-pound player was handed the football. I knew as soon as I saw him with the ball in hand and a full head of steam moving directly toward me that this tackle was going to hurt. I was significantly undersized (as I was for all my sports participations). I did my best to aim low (I was short so that part was easy), and wrap his legs. As I attempted to do this, I felt an explosion hit my head. That explosion was his knee striking my helmet. My head hurt for several hours but the effect thankfully was very short-lived. It was a painful lesson, but a valuable one. That was my first concussion, but has endured as reminder of the cause and empathy for many of my patients' suffering.

Finally, I want to thank you, the reader. Both keeping up with advances in medicine and caring for individuals with concussions is a constant challenge. You've taken the initiative to seek out more education on the subject. Your patients will benefit greatly from your decision and dedication. As a fellow clinician, I especially admire that. As our knowledge of concussions evolves and changes, I encourage you to continue to advance your approach and care. I hope you find information in this book that will aid you in caring for your concussion patients.

Contents

About the Editor

Deepak S. Patel is board-certified in family medicine and primary care sports medicine. He practices family and sports medicine in Yorkville and Aurora, IL. He also serves as Director of Sports Medicine for Rush Copley Family Medicine Residency Program in Aurora, IL. His additional teaching affiliation is Assistant Professor at Rush Medical College, Chicago, IL.

He has served as concussion consultant for several area school districts and helped to develop their concussion policies and protocols. Dr. Patel has authored, mentored, and served as section editor for several publications and textbooks on family medicine, but more often on sports medicine topics. He has served on an evidence-based concussion working group for the American Academy of Neurology as the only primary care or sports medicine physician. He is often requested as a concussion medical expert witness for legal proceedings.

As a primary care physician, Dr. Patel is uniquely qualified to deliver education from a specialist perspective but geared toward the primary care provider. He routinely lectures on sports medicine topics at local, regional, and national CME events. One of his frequently presented topics is concussions. For several years, he has served as Chair and Subject Matter Expert on Sports Medicine and Musculoskeletal Medicine for the American Academy of Family Physician national conferences and annual FMX (AAFP Annual meeting) conference.

Dr. Patel is a Fellow of the American Academy of Family Physicians, member of the American Medical Society for Sports Medicine, and Fellow of the American College of Sports Medicine. Currently, he is also the team physician for Plano and Plainfield South High Schools. Throughout his career, he has served as team physician for high schools, Division-I Universities, and Semi-Professional sports teams.

Chapter 1
Introduction to Concussion

Deepak S. Patel

Clinical Question: An 18-year-old female falls backward and hits her head on the basketball court. Her parents are suspicious when the athletic trainer tells them she has a concussion. They ask, "How can she have a concussion when her head looks normal, she is behaving normally, and no imaging tests were performed?"

The term *concussion* is frequently used by the media, patients, and medical personnel. Concussions are a subset of *mild traumatic brain injury* (MTBI). Although these terms are often used interchangeably, many times the term MTBI is used in the literature. The challenge for providers, patients, and those around concussed individuals is that concussions often lack outward physical findings.

What Is the Definition of Concussion and How Does It Happen?

Concussion is defined by multiple international organizations as a traumatic injury to the brain that leads to a temporary impairment of brain function [1–6]. Although headache is the most common symptom, additional neurologic impairments can be demonstrated in varying severity through a number of signs and symptoms. Since some of these signs and symptoms can also occur in major traumatic brain injuries, it's important for providers to understand the differences. Most guidelines also differentiate major traumatic brain injuries from concussion by noting that concussions lack structural abnormalities on traditional imaging (CT or MRI). Commonly, the injury is not specific to direct head trauma but can even occur with indirect head

D. S. Patel (✉)
Family and Sports Medicine, Rush University Medical Center, Aurora, IL, USA
e-mail: Deepak_S_Patel@rush.edu

trauma. This indirect trauma can occur with violent head movement forward, back, or even rotationally. Such movement leads to the brain striking the inside the cranium or being rapidly shaken.

Many of these indirect brain traumas are not specific to sports or falls. Concussions occur in all age groups in various settings. Recently, more attention has been placed on sports-related concussions. Early guidelines focused on contact sports and management of athletes with concussion. However, nonathlete concussions can result from a variety of mechanisms and often have their own associated challenges. Concussions can occur in different settings such as motor vehicle accidents, on the playground, at home and at work, and in military combat. Currently, in fact, the population most well-studied on traumatic brain injuries is the military.

Regardless of the exact injury mechanism of the concussion, this type of injury leads to microscopic axonal damage. Furthermore, the stretching of axons leads to cellular and metabolic changes, which lead to alterations in ion concentrations and neurotransmitter release. The body attempts to stabilize this damage with intracellular glucose uptake to balance sodium and potassium fluxes.

As our knowledge of concussions evolves, we are faced with the challenge to define how and why concussions occur. For example, why do multiple players on the team exposed to the same brain impacts vary to such a degree in the development of concussions? Various products have been proposed to measure or dissipate head injury forces, but the specific concussion threshold for each individual varies.

Which Providers Are Best to Evaluate and Manage Concussions?

Given the frequency with which concussions occur and the diverse populations are affected, several types of providers are expected to evaluate and manage concussions. Concussion care often falls within the expertise of Neurology, Neurosurgery, Physical Medicine and Rehabilitation, and Primary Care Sports Medicine. None of these, however, specialize in concussions, and they may vary in both their experience and interest. Specialties such as Primary Care Sports Medicine and Neurology usually have the greatest experience in concussion care and have traditionally led in training physicians in concussion care. Since many concussions occur in a sporting environment, the sports medicine providers claimed greater experience in concussion care. Pediatrics, family medicine, and internal medicine providers care for concussions among their primary care patient population and often are the first providers to see patients after a concussion. In an acute setting, Emergency and Urgent Care providers regularly evaluate patients for head injuries and especially determine if a concussion or a more severe, major traumatic brain injury has occurred.

Providers in other fields have risen to meet the need of concussion care by adding specialized training and certification. Examples include neuropsychologists, neuro-optometrists, and physical therapists. Physical therapists are routinely involved in the rehabilitation needs of concussed individuals and therefore are often a valuable resource to the primary care provider.

What Is the Role of Athletic Trainers and Nurses in Evaluation and Treatment of Concussions?

Because they are present at athletic practices and games, athletic trainers are often the first providers to evaluate sports-related concussions. They are responsible for identifying when an injured athlete should seek immediate care or should be observed on the sideline. They also have direct knowledge of athletes' usual behaviors, emotional states, personalities, and tendencies, which can be invaluable when identifying changes after an injury. They provide an additional communication link between providers and coaching staff. Their close relationship with the players and team enhances an athlete's reincorporation to team practice and games. They are also well-versed in return-to-play protocols (see "Return to Play" chapter) and can supervise the exercise progression to ensure a safe return.

Nurses are also a valuable resource in concussion treatment. In a school setting, concussed students are often sent to the nurse when new or increased symptoms arise. In many school districts, nurses are responsible for administering the return-to-learn protocol and conveying any academic and physical restrictions for students. When concussed students' symptoms increase, teachers will send students to the nurse to be evaluated. In some schools, nurses will monitor student symptoms daily and convert their office into a rest location when needed.

Are There Laws Related to Concussions?

Every state in the United States now has a law related to concussion care directed at the school age concussion population. These laws vary from state to state, and the authors of this text strongly encourage each reader to consult your specific state concussion law. The laws are meant to ensure appropriate evaluation and management of concussions. The priority is to ensure that anyone suspected of having suffered a concussion is not allowed to return prematurely and be thereby placed in danger of severe complications such as second impact syndrome (see "Post-Concussion Syndrome" chapter). Many of these laws require school districts to establish policies that address individuals who may identify or interact with concussed students. Several states in the United States now require education for several school personnel such as administrators, coaches, and teachers.

Due to the impairments in daily functioning that occur, concussions can affect others around the concussed individual. It is important for family members and caregivers to be aware of the impairments and challenges that are involved with having a concussion. As you will read later in this book, communication with all supervisors or administrators is required. This can include parents, employers, teachers, school nurses, athletic trainers, and coaches.

The authors of this textbook believe that best concussion care involves communication and comprehensive attention from everyone surrounding the concussed individual.

Are There Any Good Guidelines Available for Concussion Care?

Over the years, several organizations have published and revised guidelines on concussions [1–8]. At the time of the writing of this textbook, guidelines have been available from the American Academy of Neurology, American Medical Society for Sports Medicine, Centers for Disease Control and Prevention, Parachute of Canada, Ontario Neurotrauma Foundation, and International Conference on Concussion in Sport. Each of these reflects the organization's review of literature and recommendation for care of concussed individuals. Of note, some are more specific to certain populations, and that should be considered when reviewing those guidelines.

Where Can Patients Find Reliable Information About Concussions?

Although our understanding and management of concussions continue to evolve, providers and patients may need to search for additional resources. The resources may provide patients and parents further information on concussion background, warning signs, general restrictions, and recovery process. Although generic and not specific to every concussed individual, this can be a helpful addition to information and care conveyed by medical providers. Providers should remind patients that each concussion is unique and therefore the care and expectations should be individualized.

These resources may also be required by providers to consider updated information or specific resources for patients and the community. Several websites contain excellent information about concussions. Some suggestions at the time of publication of this text include:

- American Academy of Family Physicians: http://www.aafp.org/patient-care/ public-health/sports-medicine/concussions.html
- American Medical Society for Sports Medicine: https://journals.lww.com/cjs-portsmed/Fulltext/2016/09000/AMSSM_Position_Statement_on_Cardio-vascular.1

- Brain Injury Guidelines - Ontario Neurotrauma Foundation (ONF): https://brain-injuryguidelines.org/
- Center for Disease Control and Prevention (CDC): http://www.cdc.gov/headsup/providers/
- Child SCAT6: https://bjsm.bmj.com/content/bjsports/57/11/636.full.pdf
- Child SCOAT 6 (> 3 day post injury): https://bjsm.bmj.com/content/bjsports/57/11/672/DC1/embed/inline-supplementary-material-1.pdf?download=true
- Concussion recognition tool (CRT) 6: https://bjsm.bmj.com/content/bjsports/57/11/692.full.pdf
- Consensus statement on concussion in sport: the 6th International Conference on Concussion in Sport: https://bjsm.bmj.com/content/57/11/695.long
- Ontario Neuro Trauma Foundation: https://onf.org/3rd-edition-guidelines-for-concussion-mild-traumatic-brain-injury-and-persistent-symptoms/
- Parachute Canada: http://www.parachutecanada.org/home/print/2346/
- SCAT 6: https://bjsm.bmj.com/content/bjsports/57/11/622.full.pdf
- SCOAT 6: https://bjsm.bmj.com/content/bjsports/57/11/651.full.pdf
- Team Physician: https://bjsm.bmj.com/content/early/2021/06/23/bjsports-2021-104235

Key Points
- Concussion is a type of mild traumatic brain injury (MTBI) that leads to temporary neurologic impairment.
- Several different medical specialties are involved in concussion care.
- Consult appropriate state laws related to concussions especially regarding children and students.
- Several different guidelines and websites may add additional information for both patients and providers.

References

1. Herring S, Kibler WB, Putukian M, et al. Selected issues in sport-related concussion (SRC|mild traumatic brain injury) for the team physician: a consensus statement. BJSM. 2021; https://doi.org/10.1136/bjsports-2021-104235.
2. Corwin DJ, Grady MF, Master CL, Joffe MD, Zonfrillo MR. Evaluation and management of pediatric concussion in the acute setting. Pediatr Emerg Care. 2021;37(7):371–9.
3. Rose SC, Anderson W, Feinberg D, Ganesh A, Green L, Jaffee M, Kaplen M, Lorincz M, De Luigi A, Patel D, Tsao JW, Lee E, Webb A. Quality improvement in neurology concussion quality measurement set. Neurology. 2021;97(11):537–42. https://doi.org/10.1212/WNL.0000000000012537.
4. Podolak OE, Arbogast KB, Master CL, Sleet D, Grady MF. Pediatric sports-related concussion: an approach to care. Am J Lifestyle Med. 2022;16(4):469–84. https://doi.org/10.1177/1559827620984995.
5. Patricios JS, Schneider KJ, Dvorak J, Ahmed OH, Blauwet C, Cantu RC, Davis GA, Echemendia RJ, Makdissi M, McNamee M, Broglio S. Consensus statement on concussion in sport: the 6th International Conference on Concussion in Sport–Amsterdam, October 2022. Br J Sports Med. 2023;57(11):695–711.

6. Echemendia RJ, Burma JS, Bruce JM, et al. Acute evaluation of sport-related concussion and implications for the Sport Concussion Assessment Tool (SCAT6) for adults, adolescents and children: a systematic review. BJSM. 2023;57:722–35.
7. Patricios JS, et al. Beyond acute concussion assessment to office management: a systematic review informing the development of a Sport Concussion Office Assessment Tool (SCOAT6) for adults and children. Br J Sports Med. 2023;57(11):737–48.
8. Davis GA, et al. Pediatric sport-related concussion: recommendations from the Amsterdam consensus statement 2023. Pediatrics. 2024;153:1.

Chapter 2
Incidence and Risk Factors for Concussions

Deepak S. Patel, Elizabeth Yucknut, and Natasha Ahmed

Case: A 15-year-old female soccer player sustained a concussion 10 days ago after a collision, resulting in temporary disorientation but no loss of consciousness or amnesia. She has been following her physician's advice to rest and limit physical activity but continues to experience lingering fatigue, difficulty concentrating, and occasional headaches. Her father is worried about the duration of her recovery and would like to know the chances of his daughter experiencing another concussion in the future.

In her age group, most concussions are related to sports, with soccer having one of the highest incidence rates among females. Having already experienced one concussion increases her risk of sustaining another. While no outcome can be guaranteed, it is important for the physician to inform the father that her risk of a subsequent concussion is higher compared to many of her peers.

Question: Are concussions becoming more common?

Concussion is a widespread form of trauma experienced among all populations regardless of age, race, gender, or mechanism of injury. Strong epidemiological framework is important for understanding the nature of mTBIs. As we will see later in this section, age, sex, and mechanism of injury-related patterns are relevant when comparing incidence rates. There is thought to be an underestimation considering the number of unreported injuries [1–5]. For example, data collected from hospitals and emergency rooms do not account for injuries seen in outpatient settings and organized sports settings with athletic trainers. The World Health Organization (WHO) estimates a true incidence exceeding 600 per 100,000 people each year [6].

At a global level, there is a one in five lifetime risk of concussion [7]. Mild TBI-related emergency department visit rates increased from 2006 to 2012 across all age

D. S. Patel (✉)
Family and Sports Medicine, Rush University Medical Center, Aurora, IL, USA
e-mail: deepak_S_patel@rush.edu

E. Yucknut · N. Ahmed
Rush Medical College, Chicago, IL, USA

groups and gender [1, 2, 8]. The highest rates are seen in both male and female between the ages of 0 and 4 years, 15 and 24 years, and elderly females over the age of 65 years [8].

Each year, 1.6 to 3.8 million concussions are estimated to result from sports/recreational injuries in the United States [9, 10]. Fortunately, as seen in Fig. 2.1, the rate of ED visits each year among children for sports and recreation-related TBI decreased by 27% in 2012–2018 [11]. In the United States, there are almost eight million athletes participating in high school athletics and almost 500,000 student athletes competing within the National Collegiate Athletic Association (NCAA) [12]. Concussions represent 14.8% of sports-related injuries in high school, being the second most common injury after ankle strain/sprain, and 5.8–6.2% of collegiate injuries [12, 13]. The increases in trends are thought to be multifactorial. It can be hypothesized that parents, players, coaches, and the general public are more aware of the seriousness and complications of these injuries leading to increased sensitivity in reporting these injuries [14, 15].

Sports-Related Concussions

Question: What are the risk factors associated with higher concussions rates in athletes?

There is a well-established understanding of increased risk with individuals having a history of previous concussions [16, 17]. Marshall et al. [18] found that athletes with a history of one concussion in the last 2 years had over two times the rate of concussion, and those with two or more prior concussions had up to five times higher rate when compared to individuals with no history of prior concussion. Furthermore, high school students who played on multiple sports teams were found to have positive correlation with the number of reported concussions. Athletes who played on one to three sports teams increased their concussion incidence from 16.7, 22.9, and 30.5%, respectively [3].

Certain positions and actions in specific sports increase the risk for concussions. In high school football and rugby, the majority of concussions are from tackling or being tackled [13, 19]. A 2021 study funded by the Centers for Disease Control and Prevention (CDC) showed that tackle football athletes sustained a greater number of head impacts per AE (athletic exposure) and were at increased risk for high-magnitude impacts compared with flag football athletes aged 6–14 years old [20]. Heading the ball is a risk factor in both boys and girls soccer. In girls' volleyball, digging accounts for over one-third of concussions, while takedowns account for more than half of concussions in boys' wrestling [13].

Question: When in sports do concussions typically occur?

Current evidence has started to reveal a few trends in terms of timing of SRCs. One of these trends being that concussions have been shown to occur more often in

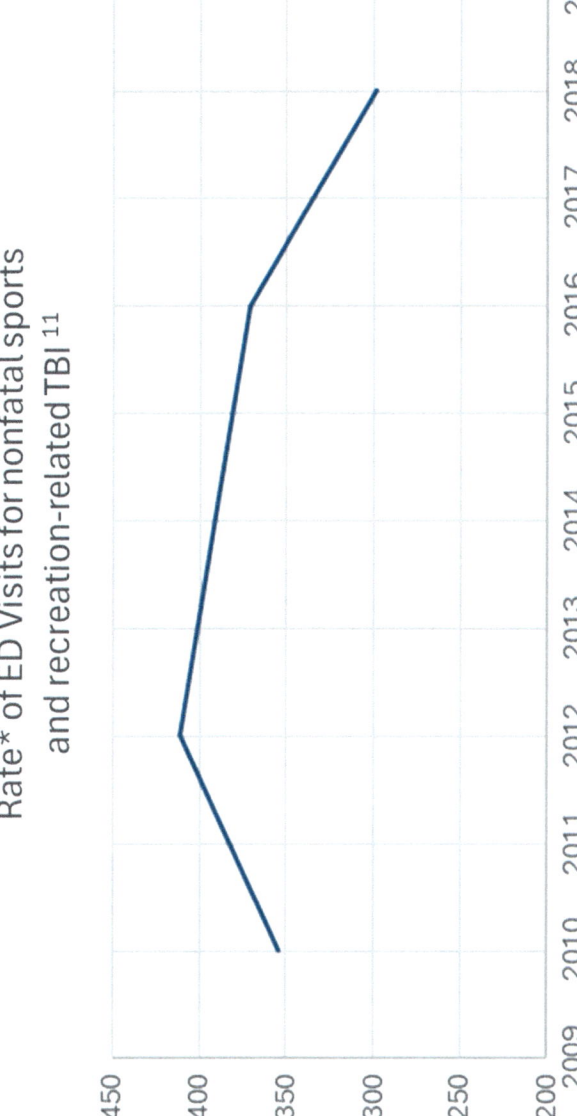

Fig. 2.1 Rate* of ED visits for nonfatal sports and recreation-related TBI^11. * Per 100,000 population

games as opposed to practice [12, 13, 19, 21, 22]. In a meta-analysis including 83 studies of high school and college athletes from 2001 to 2019, games were associated with 2.01 more concussions per 10,000 AEs than practice, with the greatest difference between games and practices observed with football, ice hockey, and rugby [12]. A 2019 study including 20 high school sports during 2013–2014 to 2017–2018 school years showed that 63.7% of reported concussions occurred during competition [21]. Additionally on the high school level, the most recent data from reporting information online (RIO) concluded that concussions accounted for 18% of injuries during competition, while concussions accounted for 11% of injuries during practice [13]. The majority of sports in the 2022–2023 school year had a higher percentage of SRCs in competition as opposed to practice, with the two exceptions being boys' basketball and baseball (Fig. 2.2). This was seen again in a 2-year cohort of female and male high school rugby players. There were 429 injuries recorded, with 113 being a concussion during a match, and only 29 recorded as a concussion during a training session [19]. Chandran et al. had a similar conclusion from a collegiate level, with SRC incidence being consistently higher in competition compared to practice for men's and women's sports. The most markedly differential incidence was seen in men's hockey, with a competition SRC rate of 23.36 per 10,000 AEs and only 1.77 in practice [22]. The lesser incidence in practice could be attributable to protective features and adaptations to player drills intended to reduce the frequency of contact [22].

Additionally, studies have shown that concussions during a game are more likely to occur in the later half of the game. Most concussions sustained during practice occur after the first hour. Similarly, the majority of concussions sustained during competition occur in the second half or third/fourth quarter [21]. It has also been shown that concussions are more likely to occur while in season as opposed to off

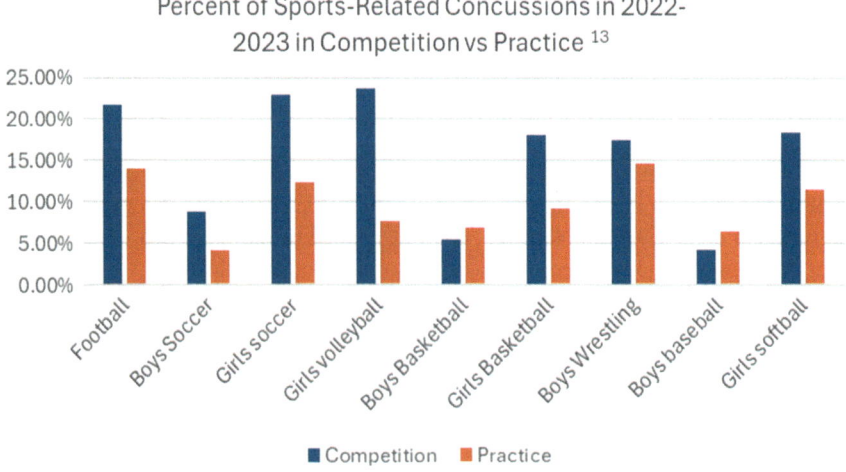

Fig. 2.2 Percent of sports-related concussions in 2022-2023 in competition vs practice^13

season. A large majority of concussions are sustained during the regular season, followed by preseason, and then postseason [21, 22].

Children and Adolescent Age Groups

Question: Are concussions more common in older or younger children?

All age groups are at risk for experiencing mild traumatic brain injury (mTBI). It is estimated that about 50% of concussions sustained in North America annually come from the children/adolescent age group [7]. Concussion experiences were found to vary by demographic as there are significant misconceptions regarding the causes, symptoms, recovery course, and risks.

Children under the age of 18 years made up an average of 283,000 ED visits from 2001 to 2016 with highest rates between 10 and 17 years old [11]. In 2022, the CDC reported that 2.3 million children and adolescents aged ≤17 years had ever received a diagnosis of a concussion or brain injury. Diagnosis of a concussion or brain injury increased with age, from 1.0% among those aged 0–5 years to 2.3% among those aged 6–11 years and 5.9% among those aged 12–17 years [23].

When comparing high school and collegiate athletes, studies have shown that collegiate athletes have a higher concussion rate. A meta-analysis from 2001 to 2019 concluded an overall concussion rate for high school sports to be 3.66 per 10,000 AEs, compared to 3.78 concussions per 10,000 AEs in college sports [12].

Question: Are concussions in children more common from sports or accidents?

It has been estimated that 36–60% of concussions in children and adolescents are sports-related [7]. According to the most recent CDC analysis, using the National Electronic Injury Surveillance System All Injury Program (NEISS-AIP) found that across a 7-year study period, approximately 2 million children sustained head injuries due to sports- or recreational-related activities [24]. The majority of concussions in the child and adolescents under the age of 18 are caused by sports- and recreational-related activities such as injuries occurring in football, soccer, basketball, wrestling, bicycling, roller-skating, bicycling, and playground activities [24, 25]. Historically, sports-related concussions have been a primary focus, while newer studies are starting to examine concussion incidence in a variety of settings beyond sports. Yaramothu et al. conducted a study examining the incidence of a large pediatric concussion population in a broad range of daily activities. As depicted in Fig. 2.3, concussions were most prevalent in organized sports, followed by injuries in school settings including PE, recreational activities, motor vehicle collisions, and lastly at home [26]. Concussion rates have been found to increase with age, predominately in older children 10–14 years old and adolescents aged 15–17 years old with contact sports being twice as common when compared to noncontact sports and four times when compared to recreational activities [24]. High school football

Concussion Incidence in Pediatric Population [26]

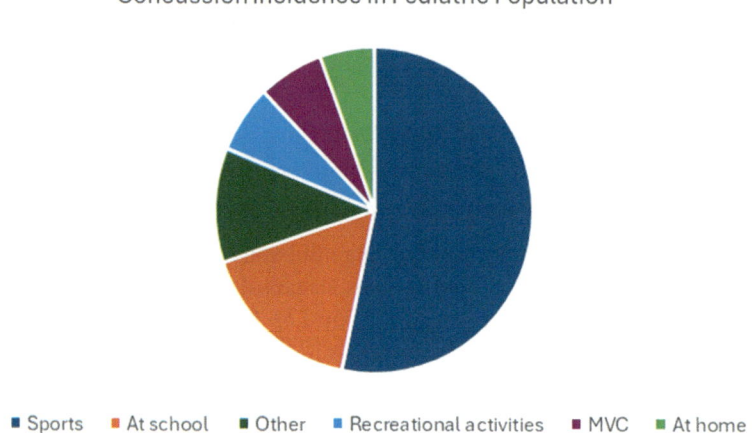

■ Sports   ■ At school   ■ Other   ■ Recreational activities   ■ MVC   ■ At home

Fig. 2.3 Concussion incidence in pediatric population^26

is the most well-studied cohort for adolescents, whereas data for the younger age group is not as well studied.

High School

Question: High School football is regularly identified to be associated with concussions, but are there other sports that also have a high incidence?

Nearly 8 million high school students participate in organized sports, making a large portion of the athletes at risk for SRC [15]. National survey of high school students identified that over 50% of students between the ages of 15 and 19 years old have played on at least one sports team with greater than 64% seen in males [25]. The high school reporting information online (RIO) reported an overall injury rate of 2.41 in the 2022–2023 school year, with 14.8% of injuries being concussions. Concussion was the most common type of injury in football, girls' soccer, boys' wrestling, and girls' softball. Concussion was the second most common type of injury for boys' and girls' basketball, as well as girls' volleyball, with ankle strain/sprain being the most common [13]. Although a less commonly played sport in the United States, Rugby is currently classified as the sport with the highest concussion rate [12]. Rugby is typically not included in the research studies analyzing concussion rates within the United States. In such studies, American football typically has the highest concussion rate [21, 27]. The SRC rate for American football is greater in high school compared to college [12].

Question: Although males and females may play similar sports, do their concussion rates vary?

Multiple large-scale studies conclude males are 1.4 times more likely to sustain head injuries in non-sports-related settings as compared to females. However, in gender-comparable sports such as soccer, females have the highest rate of injury, notably concussions (Fig. 2.4) [12, 19, 28]. Van Pelt et al. described a greater concussion rate in females for the majority of gender-comparable sports, with one exception being males having a greater concussion rate than females in lacrosse [12]. Furthermore, Shill et al. observed high school rugby players had a 70% higher concussion rate than males [19]. For US high schools in the 2022–2023 school year, girls were 2.71 times more likely to sustain a concussion compared to boys in soccer. There were similar findings in basketball and softball/baseball, with relative risk for girls being 2.46 and 2.77, respectively [13].

There are several potential reasons why female student-athletes may incur SRCs more often than males. Females have a decreased head-neck segment mass, neck girth, and strength compared with males, which may predispose them to have greater linear and angular acceleration [28]. Additionally, some studies have shown that females are more willing to disclose their SRC compared with males [29]. Commonly, male athletes more than females may try to conceal their symptoms from coaches or medical staff hoping to avoid losing playing time. This may be driven by societal pressures, fear of being sidelined, or a desire to maintain their position on the team [28].

There has also been evidence to show sex-based differences at the high school and collegiate level in terms of mechanism of injury. Males have shown to have a higher number of concussions due to contact with another person, while females have more concussions due to contact with equipment or an apparatus [21, 22]. Bretzin et al.'s analysis of sex differences in SRCs in high school student athletes for the 2015–2016 academic school year revealed significant differences between sexes for time loss in returning to sport. The mean number of days from injury to authorized date of return to sport was 13.8 for females, as opposed to 12.0 in males.

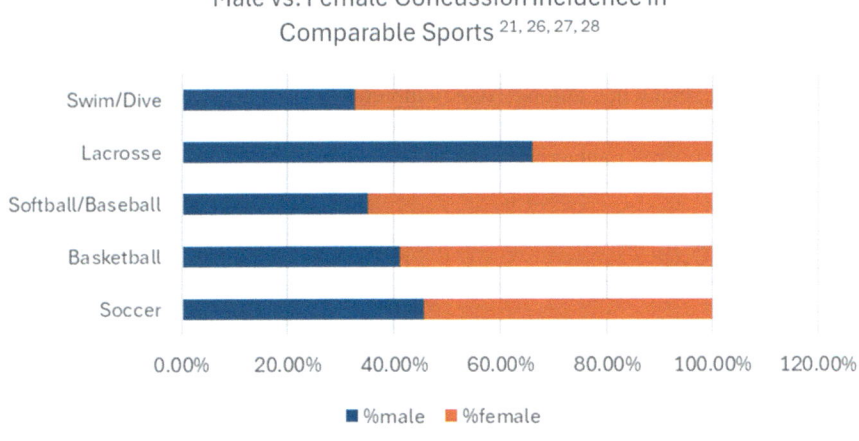

Fig. 2.4 Male vs. Female concussion incidence in comparable sports^21, 26, 27, 28

Bretzin et al. additionally analyzed numbers of missed school days but found no significant difference between sexes [28].

Collegiate Sports

Question: Are rates of SRC less common in college sports?

According to the National College Athletic Association (NCAA), 460,000 athletes participate in collegiate sports annually, making this a population at high risk for developing sports-related concussions [30]. Overall, collegiate athletes have been found to have higher concussion rates than high school athletes [12]. The NCAA Injury Surveillance Program (ISP) uses a convenience sample of varsity NCAA athletes from 25 championship sports during the 2014/2015 through 2018/2019 academic years and found an overall SRC rate of 4.13 per 10,000 AE [22]. Highest rates were seen in men's ice hockey, followed by women's soccer, women's ice hockey, and men's football. This study focuses on NCAA sports but does not account for popular full contact club sports such as rugby. A prospective study comparing collegiate rugby to football found a significant rate difference in concussions with 2.5 in rugby versus 1.0 in football and a significantly higher incidence occurring during games over practice sessions [31]. There have been several changes in NCAA sports in terms of gameplay rules as well as SRC evaluation and management in recent years. In an effort to decrease the rate of SRC, the NCAA instituted the "targeting" rule which was a personal foul defined as initiating contact with the crown of a helmet or targeting a defenseless player in the head and neck area. In 2013, this rule was expanded by the violation of rule not only being a personal foul but additionally an automatic ejection from the game [32]. Established in 2018 and updated in January 2024, the NCAA established the Concussion Safety Advisory Group who created a concussion safety protocol checklist for colleges, most recently updated in January 2024. This checklist supports schools' compliance with concussion protocol management legislation and serves as a guide for professionals managing concussion sustained by college athletes [33]. Further investigations into SRC incidence among NCAA athletes will be critical in the upcoming years to understand if these changes were effective in reducing rates of concussions and improving overall concussion care.

Professional Sports

Question: We hear about professional players with concussions in the public media, but what is their incidence?

The National Football League (NFL) has been in the spotlight for almost two decades for its criticism regarding player safety after sustaining traumatic brain injuries, leading to changes in management policies, and penalties for aggressive play [34]. From 2002 to 2015, NFL surveillance data showed a steady increase in concussion rates. There was an overall incidence per game of 0.38 in 2002–2007, followed by .658 in 2010–2014, and then lastly .715 in 2015 [35]. After 2015, concussion rates started to decrease annually, with an incidence per game in 2019 of 0.531 [35]. At the start of the 2018–2019 season, a new rule called "article 8" was introduced. This rule expanded the helmet-hit regulations, making it a foul for a player to lower their head and initiate contact with an opponent using their helmet. If a player is in violation of the rule, the team is penalized 15 yards and subject to possible disqualification from the game pending replay review. Baker et al. analyzed NFL players placed on publicly available injury reports for a concussion from 2016–2017 to 2019–2020 and found a 40% decrease in SRC rate when comparing the post-article 8 cohort to pre-article 8 cohort [32]. Recent data suggests no difference in injuries due to helmet-body collisions versus helmet-helmet and helmet-surface injuries [34]. A concussion is reported almost every other game in the NFL, but this number is likely to be higher due to underreporting [34, 35]. This rise in incidence established a precedent for implementing safety standards. However, the increase may also be attributed to frequent changes in management policies.

Military

Question: Do military personnel have higher rates of concussions compared to civilians?

Since the conflicts in Afghanistan and Iraq, traumatic brain injuries have gained attention among military service members between 18 and 24 years old. Over 80% of traumatic brain injuries are classified as mTBI in deployed and non-deployed settings [36]. There has been an estimated 283% increase in concussion rate in military service members from 2000 to 2011 [6]. The Department of Defense (DoD) has implemented its own surveillance data and policies to address these injuries [6]. Although many of the principles overlap with the demographics already discussed above, there are several unique factors that are specific to this group such as mechanism of injury, comorbidities, and military culture. The US military identifies with a culture that has its own set of values such as selfless service and mission focus over personal needs. This may affect the way these injuries are identified and managed when compared to the civilian population. These values also predispose them to recurrent injury. Non-deployed service members are also engaged in physically demanding training activities, motor vehicle crashes, sporting, and recreational events [6]. Psychiatric comorbidities such as post-traumatic stress disorder (PTSD) commonly seen in service members include symptoms such as sleep, mood, and cognitive disturbances [6]. Data for deployed men is difficult to attain and is not included in DoD reports. According to survey data, the most common cause of TBI is contributed to blast injuries, motor vehicle accidents, and falls. Given the context in which blast injuries occur, it is difficult to quickly identify and manage concussions from blast injuries in an acute setting and further research is warranted.

General Adult Population

Question: What are other common causes of concussions excluding sports or military involvement?

In a self-reported asking adults who sustained a concussion the mechanism of their injury, 24% reported being struck by or against something by accident, 21.2% reported falling or tripping, 15.4% reported being involved in a motor vehicle crash, 5.9% reported being struck by or against something during a fight or argument, 4.9% reported riding a bicycle, and the remainder reported "other" [5]. These findings are very similar to a report from the CDC that reviewed TBI-related ED visits from 2007 to 2013. The CDC concluded that in the general population, including both adults and children, falls are the leading cause of concussions, followed by being struck by an object or against an object and motor vehicle crashes [37]. Among females older than 65 years old, the third highest annual rate of mTBI is observed, often accompanied by comorbidities such as diabetes, poly-pharmacy, and age-related changes (e.g., hearing, vision, strength, balance, cognitive function). Increasing fall risk predisposes this age group to sustain head injuries with prolonged recovery [6]. Consequently, it is reasonable to expect the elderly population to have a high incidence of mTBI. However, due to the multiple comorbidities mentioned, these conditions may take precedence during acute management.

Comorbid Neuropsychological Conditions

Question: What medical conditions predispose or complicate the management of concussions?

The prevalence of attention deficit hyperactivity disorder (ADHD) is associated with increased cognitive deficits and reporting of concussion-type symptoms [6]. The American Medical Society for Sports Medicine consensus statement classifies ADHD as a "concussion modifier," such that it is associated with increased cognitive dysfunction and prolongs recovery [17]. Similarly, small-scale studies have identified challenges of diagnosis and management of concussions with comorbid conditions such as anxiety, depression, and PTSD [38]. Symptoms of these conditions such as fatigue, difficulty to concentrate, memory impairment, and sleep disturbances often overlap with concussion symptoms. Optimizing these underlying conditions is important in the recovery of mTBI as these untreated conditions also are thought to contribute to persistence of concussion-like symptoms. Alcohol is not included in any large studies and has predominantly been studied in the setting of severe traumatic brain injuries, rather than in mTBI. However, in the ED about one third to a quarter of patients with recreational head injuries had an elevated blood alcohol concentration [25]. One study attributed an inverse relationship with young male adults of lower socioeconomic status with alcohol use and physical assault leading to injuries including concussions [8]. The effects of alcohol including impaired motor control, lack of inhibition, and heightened risk-taking behaviors predispose predominantly younger males to violence and falls [38].

Future Data

Question: Is there a way to more accurately report concussion rates in the future?

Current data sources may only capture one out of every nine concussions across the nation [39]. The majority of current reputable surveillance systems reporting traumatic brain injuries rely on hospital-based data sets, more particularly within emergency rooms [4]. These surveillance systems neglect to account for the number of TBIs that were identified in outpatient settings or by athletic trainers, as well as the number of individuals with TBIs that did not seek medical attention. A national study performed in 2018 asked 10,904 US adults 18 years or older to complete a questionnaire about sustaining particular injuries in their lifetime, with 1,835 adults self-reported sustaining a concussion during their lifetime. Of those individuals, 50.4% were never evaluated by a doctor or nurse, with a higher proportion of these individuals being male (56.8%) [5]. It was recommended by the 2014 National Academy of Science Engineering and Medicine that the Centers for Disease Control and Prevention (CDC) creates a national surveillance system that would more accurately determine incidence sports and recreation-related TBI [4]. The Traumatic Brain Injury Program Reauthorization Act of 2018 was signed into law on December 21, 2018, which allows the CDC to implement the National Concussion Surveillance System (NCSS). The CDC finished a pilot test in fall of 2019 which involved using a self-report survey to collect TBI data [39]. The main goals of the NCSS include more insight into the main causes of concussion that are non-sports-related, providing national estimates into sports-related concussions both in and outside of organized sports, closer tracking of annual rates to see if implemented prevention strategies are effective, and providing a better understanding about where patients seek care for concussions [39].

Key Points
- Rate of contact sports-related mTBI ED visits is starting to decline.
- Higher risk of injury during competition versus practice.
- Male football players have the highest rate of concussion in the United States.
- Male rugby players have the highest rate of concussion internationally.
- In gender-comparable sports, female soccer players have the highest rate of concussions.

- Adolescent age groups have higher incidence of contact SRC as compared to noncontact sports.
- Prior concussion and playing on multiple sports teams have a strong association with sustaining repeat concussions.
- SRC are more common in college compared to high school.
- Military have multiple risk factors due to increased physical demands, motor vehicle crashes, and exposure to blast injuries.
- Comorbid neuropsychological conditions such as depression, anxiety, PTSD, ADHD, or being under the influence of alcohol may complicate the diagnosis and recovery of concussions.
- The CDC will be implementing the National Concussion Surveillance System (NCSS) in an effort to improve underreporting of concussions.

References

1. Rose SC, Weber KD, Collen JB, Heyer GL. The diagnosis and management of concussion in children and adolescents. Pediatr Neurol. 2015;53(2):108–18.
2. Voss JD, Connolly J, Schwab KA, Scher AI. Update on the epidemiology of concussion/mild traumatic brain injury. Curr Pain Headache Rep. 2015;19(7):32.
3. DePadilla L, Miller GF, Jones SE, Peterson AB, Breiding MJ. Self-Reported concussions from playing a sport or being physically active among high school students – United States, 2017. Morb Mortal Wkly Rep. 2018;67:682–5.
4. Daugherty J, Peterson A, Waltzman D, Breiding M, Chen J, Xu L, DePadilla L, Corrigan JD. Rationale for the development of a traumatic brain injury case definition for the pilot national concussion surveillance system. J Head Trauma Rehabil. 2024;39(2):115–20.
5. Womack LS, Breiding MJ, Daugherty J. Concussion evaluation patterns among US adults. J Head Trauma Rehabil. 2022;37(5):303–10.
6. Leo P, McCrea M. Epidemiology. In: Laskowitz D, Grant G, editors. Translational research in traumatic brain injury. Boca Raton: CRC Press; 2016.
7. Eliason PH, Galarneau JM, Kolstad AT, Pankow MP, West SW, Bailey S, et al. Prevention strategies and modifiable risk factors for sport-related concussions and head impacts: a systematic review and meta-analysis. Br J Sports Med. 2023;57(12):749–61.
8. Cancelliere C, Coronado VG, Taylor CA, Xu L. Epidemiology of isolated versus nonisolated mild traumatic brain injury treated in emergency departments in the United States, 2006-2012. J Head Trauma Rehabil. 2017;32(4):E37–46.
9. Hallock H, Mantwill M, Vajkoczy P, Wolfarth B, Reinsberger C, Lampit A, Finke C. Sport-related concussion: a cognitive perspective. Neurol Clin Pract. 2023;13(2):e200123.
10. American Academy of Neurology. Sports Concussion Resources. American Academy of Neurology. Accessed August 11, 2024. https://www.aan.com/practice/sports-concussion-patient-resources
11. Waltzman D, Womack LS, Thomas KE, Sarmiento K. Trends in emergency department visits for contact sports-related traumatic brain injuries among children – United States, 2001-2018. Morb Mortal Wkly Rep. 2020;69(27):870–4.
12. Van Pelt KL, Puetz T, Swallow J, et al. Data-driven risk classification of concussion rates: a systematic review and meta-analysis. Sports Med. 2021;51:1227–44.
13. Datalys Center. 2022–2023 High School RIO™ Original Summary Report. Datalys Center. Published September 2023. Accessed August 11, 2024. https://datalyscenter.org/wp-content/uploads/2023/09/2022-23-High-School-RIO-ORIGINAL-Summary-Report.pdf

14. Chen C, Shi J, Stanley RM, Sribnick EA, Groner JI, Xiang H. Trends of ED visits for pediatric traumatic brain injuries: implications for clinical trials. Int J Environ Res Public Health. 2017;14(4):E414.
15. Schallmo MS, Weiner JA, Hsu WK. Sport and sex-specific reporting trends in the epidemiology of concussions sustained by high school athletes. J Bone Joint Surg Am. 2017;99(15):1314–20.
16. Abrahams S, Mc Fie S, Patricios J, Posthumus M, September AV. Risk factors for sports concussion: an evidence-based systematic review. Br J Sports Med. 2014;48(2):91–7.
17. Harmon KG, Drezner JA, Gammons M, Guskiewicz KM, Halstead M, Herring SA, et al. American medical society for sports medicine position statement: concussion in sport. Br J Sports Med. 2013;47:15–26.
18. Marshal SW, Guskiewicz KM, Shankar V, McCrea M, Cantu RC. Epidemiology of sports-related concussion in seven US high school and collegiate sports. Inj Epidemiol. 2015;2(1):13.
19. Shill IJ, West SW, Sick S, et al. Differences in injury and concussion rates in a cohort of Canadian female and male youth Rugby Union: a step towards targeted prevention strategies. Br J Sports Med. 2024;58(1):34–41.
20. Waltzman D, Sarmiento K, Devine O, Zhang X, et al. Head impact exposures among youth tackle and flag American football athletes. Sports Health. 2021;13(5):454–62.
21. Kerr ZY, Chandran A, Nedimyer AK, et al. Concussion incidence and trends in 20 high school sports. Pediatrics. 2019;144(5):e20192180.
22. Chandran A, Boltz AJ, Morris SN, et al. Epidemiology of Concussions in National Collegiate Athletic Association (NCAA) sports: 2014/15-2018/19. AM J Sports Med. 2022;50(2):526–36.
23. QuickStats: percentage of children and adolescents aged ≤17 years who had ever received a diagnosis of concussion or brain injury, by sex and age group – national health interview survey, United States, 2022. Morb Mortal Wkly Rep 2023;72(33):899
24. Sarmiento K, Thomas KE, Daugherty J, et al. Emergency department visits for sports- and recreation-related traumatic brain injuries among children – United States, 2010–2016. Morb Mortal Wkly Rep. 2019;68:237–42.
25. Coronado VG, Haileyesus T, Cheng TA, Bell JM, Haarbauer-Krupa J, Lionbarger MR, et al. Trends in sports- and recreation-related traumatic brain injuries treated in US emergency departments. J Head Trauma Rehabil. 2015;30(3):185–97.
26. Yaramothu C, Goodman AM, Alvarez TL. Epidemiology and incidence of pediatric concussions in general aspects of life. Brain Sci. 2019;9(10):257.
27. Chun BJ, Furutani T, Oshiro R, Young C, Prentiss G, Murata N. Concussion epidemiology in youth sports: sports study of a statewide high school sports program. Sports Health. 2021;13(1):18–24.
28. Bretzin AC, Covassin T, Fox ME, et al. Sex differences in the clinical incidence of concussions, missed school days, and time loss in high school student-athletes: part 1. AM J Sports Med. 2018;46(9):2263–9.
29. Cheng J, Ammerman B, Santiago K, et al. Sex-based differences in the incidence of sports-related concussion: systematic review and meta-analysis. Sports Health. 2019;11(6):486–91.
30. Kerr ZY, Roos KG, Djoko A, Dalton SL, Broglio SP, Marshall SW, et al. Epidemiologic measures for quantifying the incidence of concussion in national collegiate athletic association sports. J Athl Train. 2017;52(3):167–74.
31. Willigenburg NW, Borchers JR, Quincy R, Kaeding CC, Hewett TE. Comparison of injuries in American collegiate football and club rugby. Am J Sports Med. 2016;44:753–60.
32. Baker HP, Lee CS, Qin C, Fibranz C, Rizzi A, Athiviraham A. Playing rule article eight decreases the rate of sport related concussion in NFL players over two seasons. Phys Sportsmed. 2021;49(3):342–7.
33. NCAA. Concussion safety protocol management. NCAA. Accessed August 11, 2024. https://www.ncaa.org/sports/2016/7/20/concussion-safety-protocol-management.aspx
34. Yengo-Kahn AM, Johnson DJ, Zuckerman SL, Solomon GS. Concussions in the national football league: a current concepts review. Am J Sports Med. 2016;44(3):801–11.

35. Mack CD, Solomon G, Covassin T, Theodore N, Cárdenas J, Sills A. Epidemiology of concussion in the national football league, 2015-2019. Sports Health. 2021;13(5):423–30.
36. Armistead-Jehle P, Soble JR, Cooper DB, Belanger HG. Unique aspects of traumatic brain injury in military and veteran populations. Phys Med Rehabil Clin N Am. 2017;28(2):323–37.
37. Taylor CA, Bell JM, Breiding MJ, Xu L. Traumatic brain injury–related emergency department visits, hospitalizations, and deaths – United States, 2007 and 2013. MMWR Surveill Summ. 2017;66(SS-9):1–16.
38. Scheenen ME, de Koning ME, van der Horn HJ, Roks G, Yilmaz T, van der Naalt J, et al. Acute alcohol intoxication in patients with mild traumatic brain injury: characteristics, recovery, and outcome. J Neurotrauma. 2016;33(4):339–45.
39. Centers for Disease Control and Prevention. Traumatic Brain Injury Programs. Centers for Disease Control and Prevention. Accessed August 11, 2024. https://www.cdc.gov/traumatic-brain-injury/programs/?CDC_AAref_Val=https://www.cdc.gov/traumaticbraininjury/research-programs/ncss/index.html

Chapter 3
Signs and Symptoms of Concussion

LaRae L. Seemann and George G. A. Pujalte

Clinical Case

A 12-year-old female presents to the clinic with her parents for a well-child visit. She plays soccer for the local team. Her parents are concerned that she might develop a concussion through heading a soccer ball or by colliding with another player. They also want to know what signs and symptoms they should be aware of to suspect that their child might have sustained a concussion.

The diagnosis of concussion can be elusive and continues to be a challenge for primary care providers. Despite the public interest and plethora of research on the pathophysiology, diagnosis, and management of concussions, there remains a lot of mystery. Every year, the number of cases of concussion and the detrimental consequences of misdiagnoses continue to rise. Primary care providers are often the first to assess a concussed patient and are therefore well-positioned in the healthcare system to diagnose, treat, and prevent concussions and its sequelae. It is imperative for primary care providers to be aware of the constellation of signs and symptoms that present with a concussion.

Question: What are the six domains of signs and symptoms of concussions?

The American Medical Society for Sports Medicine's most recent position statement on concussions divides the signs and symptoms of concussions into six domains [1]. Many of the symptoms of concussion are general and can overlap domains. The six domains with their symptoms are listed in Table 3.1.

L. L. Seemann
Primary Care Sports Medicine, University of Florida, Gainesville, FL, USA

G. G. A. Pujalte (✉)
Departments of Family Medicine, and Orthopedics and Sports Medicine, Mayo Clinic, Jacksonville, FL, USA
e-mail: Pujalte.George@mayo.edu

© The Author(s), under exclusive license to Springer Nature Switzerland AG 2025
D. S. Patel (ed.), *Concussion Management for Primary Care*,
https://doi.org/10.1007/978-3-031-85516-0_3

Table 3.1 Domains and symptoms

Domains	Examples
Headache-migraine	Headache, nausea, photosensitivity, neck pain, phonophobia, photophobia
Cognitive	Confusion, disorientation, inattention, mental fogginess, slurred speech, vacant stare
Anxiety-mood	Agitation, flat effect, depression, labile mood, anxiety
Ocular	Blurry vision, double vision, eye fatigue
Fatigue	Tiredness, decreased arousal, somnolence, difficulty sleeping
Vestibular	Imbalance, abnormal visual motion sensitivity

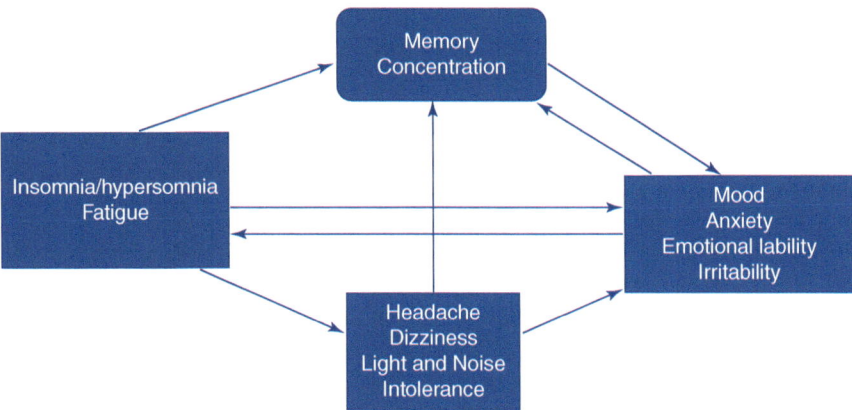

Fig. 3.1 Symptoms in one category of a concussion can interact to exacerbate symptoms in a different category [3]

Most signs and symptoms are gathered from retrospective recall studies, with a few studies using video evidence. Examples of video signs of concussion include lying motionless for greater than 2 min, motor incoordination, impact seizures, tonic posturing, and blank or vacant look [2]. It is important to note that the signs and symptoms of concussions are often very general and easy to overlook. Many signs and symptoms can also overlap into multiple categories, or a symptom in one category can compound symptoms of another category, as seen in Fig. 3.1. It is also important to clearly define symptoms that patients report. Many words to describe the symptoms are generalizable and can mean several different things, such as dizziness or confusion. Knowing exactly what patients are experiencing is necessary, as it could help guide which domain the problem fits into and the rehabilitation required.

Another important aspect when assessing concussion symptoms is to compare to a patient's baseline. A patient may have a history of headaches, attention/concentration issues, or emotional lability that could be incorrectly diagnosed as a concussion symptom. This is often an obstacle for medical providers who may be meeting the patient for the first time, so it is helpful to reach out to athletic trainers, friends, or family members to get a better understanding of the athlete's personality. For example, a survey found that almost 25% of healthy, non-concussed children reported difficulty with concentration [4]. Athletes with a concussion history also reported greater physical, emotional, and sleep-related symptoms at baseline than those with no history of concussion [5]. A wrongly diagnosed concussion-related symptom could delay a patient's return to school and sports.

The physical symptoms associated with concussions are sometimes the most obvious to the patient and family members, especially immediately after the concussion occurs [6]. Patients and family members are more likely to recognize and report many of the physical symptoms to providers, as compared to complaints in other domains [6]. However, some studies indicate that up to 25% of youth athletes think it is safe to return to play with concussion symptoms [7]. The physical signs and symptoms include headache, neck pain, drowsiness, dizziness, sensitivity to light and noise, visual and hearing changes, loss of consciousness, nausea, and vomiting [6, 7].

Signs and symptoms evolve over the subacute time period after a concussion. Furthermore, new symptoms may emerge during recovery process when the athlete starts exerting themselves. The signs and symptoms that patients experience after sustaining a concussion start in the headache-migraine and fatigue domains and progress to the anxiety-mood domain [6, 8]. Signs and symptoms in the cognitive domain can be present both early in the clinical course and months later after the trauma [6, 9]. Emotion-related sequelae of concussions more often go unrecognized, likely due to a knowledge deficit in patients and their friends and family in associating these symptoms with concussion [7].

Question: Is loss of consciousness required for a concussion?

Loss of consciousness is another often misunderstood aspect of concussions. A common public understanding is that a concussion occurred when there was a loss of consciousness. In actuality, loss of consciousness is not a requirement for diagnosing a concussion and is a somewhat rare occurrence. Only about 10% of concussions will be accompanied by a loss of consciousness [10, 11]. When loss of consciousness occurs, even for a brief period, suspicion for a concussion is extremely high, and that player should be removed from the event for evaluation at an outside facility [12]. Loss of consciousness that is prolonged (greater than 1 minute) should raise concerns of a more serious clinical presentation that requires more immediate medical attention and deviation from standard concussion protocols [13]. However, despite the severity of its presentation, there is no evidence to suggest that loss of consciousness alone is associated with more severe brain injury or worse recovery outcomes [12]. It is also essential to remember that the primary evaluation after a big hit or trauma is not to look for a concussion, more serious, possibly life-threatening, conditions need to be ruled out before worrying about concussions.

Question: What types of headache are common in patients that sustained a concussion?

Headaches are the most common complaint after a patient sustains a concussion [14, 15]. There is no specific type of headache classically associated with concussions. Headaches from concussion are usually classified as the common subtypes, with migraine and tension type predominating [16]. They are typically classified as secondary headaches. Headache prevalence, duration, and severity are greater in those with mild head injury compared with those with more severe trauma [17]. A significant number of patients have preexisting headaches, but studies conflict as to whether this is a risk factor for post-traumatic headaches [18]. Although new headaches can develop following a concussion, exacerbation of preexisting problems is likely more common [19]. If the patient has a history of migraine, then the current presentation should be compared closely with his or her typical migraine presentation. Post-traumatic headaches begin within 7 days after head trauma or after regaining consciousness. Acute headaches begin within 7 days of head trauma and may continue for up to 3 months after the injury [20].

For a small proportion of patients, the headache can persist beyond 2 months after the inciting trauma. These would be classified as chronic post-traumatic headaches and can often be severely debilitating [21]. Recurrent headaches can also be an important marker for physical or cognitive overexertion during recovery.

Neck pain, or cervicalgia, is usually included in the headache domain, as it can sometimes be the primary cause for headaches or a separate problem. It is the second most reported physical symptom of concussions [7]. Neck pain often warrants further questioning and examination to rule out other neurologic changes such as weakness, hyporeflexia, or sensory abnormalities. These findings may require a more aggressive workup with imaging and diagnostic testing [7]. It is important to keep a broad differential before concluding that a patient's neck pain is solely due to a concussion.

Referral is recommended for cervicovestibular rehabilitation if neck pain or headaches are persistent for greater than 10 days [12].

Question: What are the cognitive symptoms of concussion?

Symptoms from the cognitive domain include decreasing mental clarity, mental fogginess, difficulty concentrating, memory issues, fatigue, and confusion. Evidence demonstrates that even a single concussion can disrupt the neurological mechanisms underlying cognition [22]. Cognitive symptoms can make it difficult to assess patients for their entire constellation of symptoms. Patients are often unable to describe how they feel – this can be problematic, particularly for children and young adolescents. Concentration difficulties and memory impairment are the most common complaints in the cognitive domain [15]. Although memory impairment may be a common complaint among patients with post-concussive symptoms, the problem may involve impaired attention and concentration, forgetfulness, distractibility, slowness of mental processing and reaction time, impaired mental flexibility, working and prospective memory, and memory retrieval [23].

In the acute setting, patients can also develop post-traumatic amnesia, which affects their ability to learn new information during this period. The post-traumatic amnesia is defined as the length of time from the injury until continuous memory resumes [24]. Retrograde and anterograde post-traumatic amnesia may diminish over time with events closest to the time of trauma being most difficult to recall. Deficits of attention, working memory and recall, and executive function will likely persist long after the post-traumatic amnesia has resolved [25].

These cognitive dysfunctions can place a heavy burden on the patient and disrupt their transition back to school or work [6]. Even after the patient becomes asymptomatic, returning to their previous activities should be handled gradually. There are more cognitive challenges during this time period, which require significantly more effort and can unmask deficits that the patient previously appeared to have overcome. Memory impairment following concussion appears to involve working memory [23]. Working memory refers to the ability to temporarily store and manipulate information that is relevant for complex cognitive processes during a task [23]. The disruption of working memory impairs executive functioning and slows processing speed [23], which may present as slow responses to question or delayed recall. Fortunately, the recovery of these deficits following concussion occurs within the first weeks to months, and recovery progresses without specific intervention [24].

Question: What are the emotional or mood symptoms of concussion?

Emotional symptoms include depression, disinhibition, irritability, mood lability, depression, frustration, and restlessness. These symptoms are not typically present immediately after the injury but arise within the first week following a concussion. Self-reported changes in mood, emotions, and behavior are typically short-lived. Symptoms peak approximately 7 days after the acquisition of a concussion and resolve over a period of weeks to a month [6, 28]. It is important to talk with family members, coaches, and teammates who know the individual well, as they may notice emotional lability that is out of character. In a retrospective review of 174 concussed athletes, 50% of the sample reported at least one new emotional symptom on the Post-Concussion Symptom Scale, with the mean sub-score of emotional symptoms being 4 [28]. Additionally, a prospective cohort study found that approximately 25% of pediatric patients that were evaluated at a children's emergency department for a concussion experienced depression, irritability, or restlessness [9]. Figure 3.2 shows the neuropsychiatric symptoms that are commonly tested for in the post-concussive clinical assessment tool.

It is well-established in literature that women report higher rates of concussions compared to men [13, 30, 31]. Furthermore, females report more emotional symptoms compared to their male counterparts [4]. It has been speculated that this difference in reported symptoms of concussion was secondary to hormonal differences between males and females [32]. However, it is important to understand what baseline symptoms the patient experiences as concussion-like symptoms could have been present prior to the concussion. A systematic review and meta-analysis by Brown et al. [2] demonstrated that females report more concussion-like symptoms and emotional symptoms prior to sustaining a concussion, but the differences of these symptoms do not persist post-concussion when compared to men [33].

Female sex, along with a prior personal or family history of a psychiatry disorder, seems to be a risk factor to develop post-concussive psychiatric disorders [25].

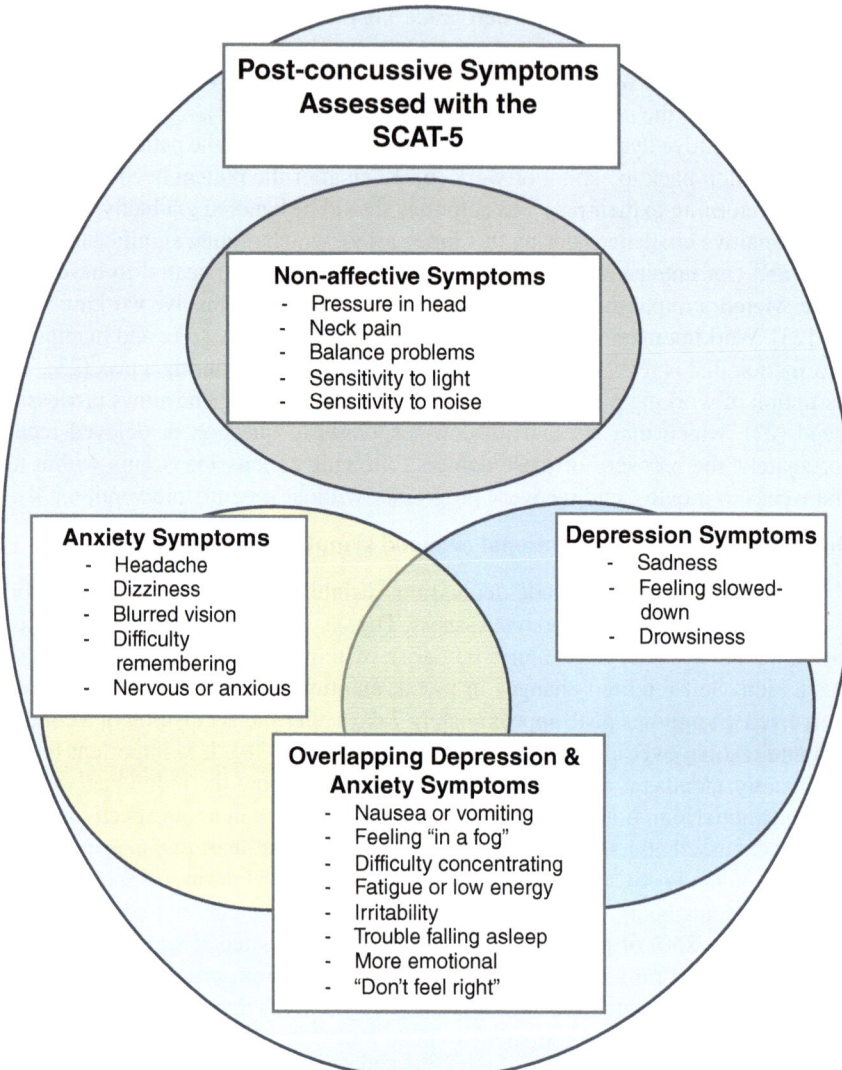

Fig. 3.2 Overlap of frequent post-concussive symptoms assessed by the Sport Concussion Assessment Tool-6 (SCAT-6). Core symptoms of mood (depression) and anxiety disorders are assessed by various psychiatric outcome measures, including the Hamilton Anxiety Scale, Beck Depression Inventory II, Generalized Anxiety Disorder-7, Brief Symptom Inventory-18, Patient Health Questionnaire-9, and the Diagnostic and Statistical Manual of Mental Disorders' (5th revision) criteria for generalized anxiety disorder and major depression. (Reprinted from Mcallister and Wall [29] with permission from Elsevier and revised to reflect SCAT-6)

Some important factors that affect the risk of developing a post-concussive psychiatric disorder are the severity of concussion injury, socioeconomic status, preinjury adaptive and intellectual functioning, and psychosocial stress [28, 34]. Personality changes secondary to the concussions is the most common post-concussive psychiatric disorders, accounting for as high as 40% of pediatric patients suffering from concussions [34, 35]. Other psychiatric disorders clinically diagnosed include depressive disorders, generalized anxiety disorder, panic disorder, post-traumatic stress disorder, obsessive-compulsive disorder, somatoform disorder, attention deficit disorder, and oppositional-defiant disorder and conduct disorder.

History of concussions is another possible risk factor for developing emotional symptoms secondary to concussion. However, it is unclear if a history of concussion predisposes people to experience more emotional symptoms or if it instead results in an increased awareness of symptoms, which, in turn, leads to increased reporting. What is known is that there exists a link between sustaining multiple concussions and long-term psychiatric and neurological disorders [36, 37] However, their association with the development of a post-concussive psychiatric disorder is undetermined [4, 28].

Concussions can cause emotional symptoms, but the diagnosis of concussion in itself can possibly affect the emotional well-being of the patient and bring out emotional symptoms. The stresses that accompany a concussion diagnosis, such as the symptoms themselves or missed school, athletics, or work, may bring out underlying mood disorders that the patient was never diagnosed with or knew they had. This may not be directly related to the concussion and therefore should not be considered a symptom that could delay rehabilitation. Nonetheless, it is imperative to understand what symptoms patients experience at baseline and be aware of the social and emotional stress that can occur with a diagnosis of a concussion.

Question: What are the ocular symptoms of concussion?

Visual deficits are more frequently being recognized and diagnosed in patients with concussions. Visual symptoms that are associated with concussions include blurry vision, double vision, and difficulty reading. Symptoms stem from a change in coordinated eye tracking, which manifests as having trouble with reading, writing, and computer-related work in school. Master, et al. (2015) found that 69% of adolescent participants had at least one visual diagnosis after a concussion and 22% had two visual diagnoses [38]. An observational study on adolescent motorcyclists found that 31% of participants reported blurry or double vision after sustaining a concussion [38].

Photophobia or light sensitivity is another common complaint in patients that sustained a concussion that can be classified in the ocular or headache-migraine domain. A third of adolescent motorcyclists previously mentioned were found to have photophobia, and one study found as high as 80% of their participants were suffering from photophobia after a concussion [15, 39]. Photophobia is usually most intense in the beginning of the clinical course and becomes less burdensome the weeks after the initial injury [6]. It is important to note that light sensitivity can be present at baseline, especially in patients that suffer from chronic migraines; therefore, it is important to clarify how their current symptoms compared to their symptoms at baseline.

Identification of concussion-related symptoms is crucial, as defects in vision can impair everyday tasks, such as driving a car, attending school, or performing work tasks, in both adults and children. Visual symptoms have high morbidity in the adolescent population because of the importance of vision to perform schoolwork activities and the increasing integration of technology within the education system. Increased screen time already causes significant visual symptoms such as eye strain and dry eyes [40], which can further be exacerbated by concussion-related visual symptoms. For this reason, improvements in clinical tools for the diagnosis and rehabilitation of visual deficits are needed.

Question: What other domain of concussion is closely related to fatigue?

Fatigue is often seen after a concussion and, like many other symptoms, can be multifactorial. Fatigue may be a primary entity, as opposed to being secondary to poor sleep. Patients often describe the fatigue as tiredness unrelated to physical or mental exertion, and sometimes it does not improve with rest. Concussion-related fatigue is usually less profound during the day than at morning or night [41]. Many athletes feel excessively sleepy and may report taking unusual daytime naps during the first week following the injury. However, napping can be disruptive to recovery and does not improve daytime sleepiness. It adversely affects the ability to fall asleep and causes less slow-wave sleep, which is viewed as most restorative [42]. Keeping a more regular day-to-day pattern of rest and activity relates to lower fatigue and depression scores [43].

After the acute phase of the injury, insomnia occurs in about 30% of people and circadian rhythm shifts in approximately 36% [44]. Several studies evaluating sleep quality post-concussion have found poor sleep quality is associated with total symptoms severity [45]. Early morning awakenings are also common and may, in turn, fuel daytime fatigue. Sleep apnea is common in post-concussion syndrome patients complaining of non-restorative sleep or waking up with headaches, and sleep apnea was associated with more memory symptoms post-concussion [46]. Females more commonly report significant sleep disturbance after sustaining a single concussion, while males may not report sleep disturbance until cumulative concussions have been sustained [47]. Reassuringly, it has been shown that 20 years post-injury, children who sustained a TBI had similar rates of being "poor sleepers" and objective outcomes across all sleep parameters when compared to a control group [48]. Fatigue can last for months after other symptoms have improved [6].

There is also a strong correlation between sleep and symptoms in other domains, especially mood. A common neurobiological mechanism may explain why concussed individuals with abnormal sleep patterns are more susceptible to depression [49]. In addition, worsening of sleep because of a concussion in those with prior history of psychiatric issues could account for increased relapses of mood symptoms and treatment resistance [50]. Several hypotheses have been proposed about the etiology of post-concussive sleep regulation and psychiatric illness including neurotransmitter imbalance, dysregulation of the hypothalamic- pituitary-adrenal axis, and genetic polymorphism, but none have been verified [51].

Question: What are the vestibular symptoms of concussion?

Vestibular symptoms are usually associated with balance alterations and dizziness, which are commonly used interchangeably. The two functional aspects of the vestibular system are the vestibulospinal component (which helps to regulate postural stability) and the vestibulo-ocular component (which integrates vision and movement of the head) [52]. Dizziness is a blanket term used by patients, which encompasses lightheadedness, blurry vision, weakness, and vertigo or unsteadiness, so it is important to get a clear description, as it could relate to different pathologies. Dizziness following concussion occurs in 50–80% of injuries [52]. Commonly tested vestibular motor symptoms include the ability to hold a tandem stance or balance on one leg. Many vestibular symptoms are evident only when provoked by stimuli or movements. Therefore, vestibular symptoms may be exacerbated by busy environments and quick head movements, such as those involved in dynamic sports or at school. Visual motion sensitivity is a phenomenon that can occur after a vestibular and/or ocular injury that refers to a heightened awareness of normal visual stimuli due to an inability to centrally integrate visual and vestibular information [52].

Balance issues can stem from the central nervous system (brain injury) or the peripheral nervous system (head injury) dysfunction [53]. Concussions can lead to balance issues also from either reason but usually from peripheral nervous system dysfunction. Some argue that vestibular symptoms may be due to a separate injury to the neck or vestibular system that occurs along with the trauma that caused the concussion. Leddy et al. found that symptom reports from patients with delayed recovery after head injury, including cognitive symptoms, do not discriminate between those with a physiologic post-concussive disorder and those with a cervical/vestibular injury [54].

Dizziness usually occurs within 72 hours after the injury, and it usually resolves within 4 to 30 days [50]. However, dizziness can last for 6 months or longer and has been implicated as a risk factor for a prolonged recovery [53]. Reported dizziness at the time of can have up to a sixfold increased rate in protracted recovery (more than 21 days), and abnormalities on vestibular-ocular reflex (VOR) testing or tandem-gait performance resulted in an average recovery time of 59 days versus just 6 days for those without vestibular abnormalities [55].

Key Points
- Concussion signs and symptoms can be broken down into six major categories: (1) vestibular, (2) ocular, (3) cognitive, (4) headache/migraine, (5) fatigue, and (6) anxiety/mood.
- Migraine and tension-type headaches are the most common types concussion headaches.
- Cognitive symptoms of concussion are decreasing mental clarity, mental fogginess, difficulty concentrating, memory issues, fatigue, and confusion.
- Emotional symptoms of concussion are depression, disinhibition, irritability, mood lability, depression, frustration, and restlessness.

- Ocular symptoms of concussion are blurry vision, double vision, and difficulty reading.
- Patients that suffer from fatigue after sustaining a concussion are likely to have emotional symptoms.
- Vestibular symptoms of concussion are balance alterations, lightheadedness, and dizziness.

References

1. Harmon KG, Clugston JR, Dec K, et al. American Medical Society for Sports Medicine position statement on concussion in sport. Clin J Sport Med. 2019;29:256.
2. Davis GA, Makdissi M, Bloomfield P, et al. International consensus definitions of video signs of concussion in professional sports. Br J Sports Med. 2019;53:1264–7.
3. Brent DA, Max J. Psychiatric sequelae of concussions. Curr Psychiatry Rep. 2017;19(12):108.
4. Hunt AW, Paniccia M, Reed N, Keightley M. Concussion-like symptoms in child and youth athletes at baseline: what is "typical"? J Athl Train. 2016;51:749–57.
5. Moser RS, Schatz P. Increased symptom reporting in young athletes based on history of previous concussions. Dev Neuropsychol. 2017;42:276–83.
6. Macartney G, Simoncic V, Goulet K, Aglipay M. Concussion symptom prevalence, severity and trajectory: implications for nursing practice. J Pediatr Nurs. 2018;40:58–62.
7. Beidler E, Bretzin AC, Schmitt AJ, Phelps A. Factors associated with parent and youth athlete concussion knowledge. J Safety Res. 2022;80:190–197.
8. Bressan S, Babl FE. Diagnosis and management of paediatric concussion. J Paediatr Child Health. 2016;52:151–7.
9. Eisenberg MA, Meehan WP, Mannix R. Duration and course of post-concussive symptoms. Pediatrics. 2014;133:999–1006.
10. Grace MT. Concussion in the pediatric patient. J Pediatr Health Care. 2013;27:377–84.
11. Halstead ME, Walter KD. Sport-related concussion in children and adolescents. Pediatrics. 2010;126:597–615.
12. Patricios JS, Schneider KJ, Dvorak J, et al. Consensus statement on concussion in sport: the 6th international conference on concussion in sport-Amsterdam, October 2022. Br J Sports Med. 2023;57(11):695-711.
13. McCrory P, Meeuwisse W, Dvorak J, et al. Consensus statement on concussion in sport—the 5th international conference on concussion in sport held in Berlin, October 2016. Br J Sports Med. 2017;51:838–47.
14. Chandran A, Elmi A, Young H, Dipietro L. Determinants of concussion diagnosis, symptomology, and resolution time in U.S. high school soccer players. Res Sports Med. 2019;1 13.
15. Harriss AB, Abbott KC, Humphreys D, Daley M, Moir ME, Woehrle E, et al. Concussion symptoms predictive of adolescent sport-related concussion injury. Clin J Sport Med. 2019; https://doi.org/10.1097/JSM.0000000000000714.
16. Bigler ED. Neuropsychology and clinical neuroscience of persistent post-concussive syndrome. J Int Neuropsychol Soc. 2008;14:1–22.
17. Couch JR, Bearss C. Chronic daily headache in the Posttrauma syndrome: relation to extent of head injury. Headache. 2001;41:559–64.
18. Jensen OK, Nielsen FF. The influence of sex and pre-traumatic headache on the incidence and severity of headache after head injury. Cephalalgia. 1990;10:285–93.
19. Choe M, Barlow KM. Pediatric traumatic brain injury and concussion. Continuum (Minneap Minn). 2018;24(1):300–11.

20. Theeler BJ, Erickson JC. Mild head trauma and chronic headaches in returning US soldiers. Headache: J Head Face Pain. 2009;49:529–34.
21. Defrin R. Chronic post-traumatic headache: clinical findings and possible mechanisms. J Man Manip Ther. 2013;22:36–44.
22. Xiong K, Zhu Y, Zhang Y, Yin Z, Zhang J, Qiu M, Zhang W. White matter integrity and cognition in mild traumatic brain injury following motor vehicle accident. Brain Res. 2014;1591:86–92.
23. Vanderploeg RD, Curtiss G, Belanger HG. Long-term neuropsychological outcomes following mild traumatic brain injury. J Int Neuropsychol Soc. 2005;11:228–36.
24. Wilson JT, Teasdale GM, Hadley DM, Wiedmann KD, Lang D. Post-traumatic amnesia: still a valuable yardstick. J Neurol Neurosurg Psychiatry. 1994;57:198–201.
25. Flynn FG. Memory impairment after mild traumatic brain injury. Continuum (Minneap Minn). 2010;16:79–109.
26. Stuss DT, Alexander MP. Executive functions and the frontal lobes: a conceptual view. Psychol Res. 2000;63(3–4):289–98.
27. Riechers RG. Rehabilitation in the patient with mild traumatic brain injury. Continuum (Minneap Minn). 2010;16:128–49.
28. Ellis MJ, Ritchie LJ, Koltek M, Hosain S, Cordingley D, Chu S, et al. Psychiatric outcomes after pediatric sports-related concussion. J Neurosurg Pediatr. 2015;16:709–18.
29. Mcallister TW, Wall R. Neuropsychiatry of sport-related concussion. Handb Clin Neurol. 2018;158:153–62.
30. Lincoln AE, Caswell SV, Almquist JL, Dunn RE, Norris JB, Hinton RY. Trends in concussion incidence in high school sports. Am J Sports Med. 2011;39:958–63.
31. Covassin T, Swanik CB, Sachs ML. Sex differences and the incidence of concussions among collegiate athletes. J Athl Train. 2003;38(3):238–44.
32. Schmelzer K, Ditzen B, Weise C, Andersson G, Hiller W, Kleinstäuber M. Clinical profiles of premenstrual experiences among women having premenstrual syndrome (PMS): affective changes predominate and relate to social and occupational functioning. Health Care Women Int. 2014;36:1104–23.
33. Brown DA, Elsass JA, Miller AJ, Reed LE, Reneker JC. Differences in symptom reporting between males and females at baseline and after a sports-related concussion: a systematic review and meta-analysis. Sports Med. 2015;45:1027–40.
34. Max JE. Neuropsychiatry of pediatric traumatic brain injury. Psychiatr Clin North Am. 2014;37:125–40.
35. Max JE, Pardo D, Hanten G, et al. Psychiatric disorders in children and adolescents six-to-twelve months after mild traumatic brain injury. J Neuropsychiatry Clin Neurosci. 2013;25:272 82.
36. Hazrati L-N, Tartaglia MC, Diamandis P, Davis KD, Green RE, Wennberg R, et al. Absence of chronic traumatic encephalopathy in retired football players with multiple concussions and neurological symptomatology. Front Hum Neurosci. 2013;7:222.
37. Lehman EJ, Hein MJ, Baron SL, Gersic CM. Neurodegenerative causes of death among retired National Football League players. Neurology. 2012;79:1970–4.
38. Master CL, Scheiman M, Gallaway M, Goodman A, Robinson RL, Master SR, Grady MF. Vision diagnoses are common after concussion in adolescents. Clin Pediatr. 2015;55:260–7.
39. Luo TD, Clarke MJ, Zimmerman AK, Quinn M, Daniels DJ, Mcintosh AL. Concussion symptoms in youth motocross riders: a prospective, observational study. J Neurosurg Pediatr. 2015;15:255–60.
40. Rosenfield M. Computer vision syndrome (a.k.a. digital eye strain). Optom Pract. 2016;17:1–10.
41. Antonioli M, Rybka J, Carvalho LA. Neuroimmune endocrine effects of antidepressants. Neuropsychiatr Dis Treat. 2012;8:65–83.
42. Centofanti SA, Dorrian J, Hilditch CJ, Banks S. Do night naps impact driving performance and daytime recovery sleep? Accid Anal Prev. 2017;99(Pt B):416–21.
43. Schmidt MH. The energy allocation function of sleep: a unifying theory of sleep, torpor, and continuous wakefulness. Neurosci Biobehav Rev. 2014;47:122–53.

44. Mosti C, Spiers MV, Kloss JD. A practical guide to evaluating sleep disturbance in concussion patients. Neurol Clin Pract. 2016;6:129–37.
45. Smulligan KL, Wilson JC, Seehusen CN, Wingerson MJ, Magliato SN, Howell DR. Post-Concussion Dizziness, Sleep Quality, and Postural Instability: A Cross-Sectional Investigation. J Athl Train. 2021;57(11-12):1072–8.
46. Santos A, Walsh H, Anssari N, Ferreira I, Tartaglia MC. Post-Concussion Syndrome and Sleep Apnea: A Retrospective Study. J Clin Med. 2020;9(3):691.
47. Oyegbile TO, Delasobera BE, Zecavati N. Gender differences in sleep symptoms after repeat concussions. Sleep Med. 2017;40:110–5.
48. Botchway EN, Godfrey C, Nicholas CL, Hearps S, Anderson V, Catroppa C. Objective sleep outcomes 20 years after traumatic brain injury in childhood. Disabil Rehabil. 2019:1–9.
49. Mollayeva T, Mollayeva S, Shapiro CM, Cassidy JD, Colantonio A. Insomnia in workers with delayed recovery from mild traumatic brain injury. Sleep Med. 2016;19:153–61.
50. Hoffer ME, Gottshall KR, Moore R, Balough BJ, Wester D. Characterizing and treating dizziness after mild head trauma. Otol Neurotol. 2004;25:135–8.
51. Mollayeva T, Mollayeva S, Colantonio A. Traumatic brain injury: sex, gender and intersecting vulnerabilities. Nat Rev Neurol. 2018;14:711–22.
52. Kontos AP, Deitrick JM, Collins MW, Mucha A. Review of vestibular and oculomotor screening and concussion rehabilitation. J Athl Train. 2017;52:256–61.
53. Mcleod TCV, Hale TD. Vestibular and balance issues following sport-related concussion. Brain Inj. 2014;29:175–84.
54. Leddy JJ, Baker JG, Merchant A, Picano J, Gaile D, Matuszak J, Willer B. Brain or strain? Symptoms alone do not distinguish physiologic concussion from cervical/vestibular injury. Clin J Sport Med. 2015;25:237–42.
55. Lau BC, Kontos AP, Collins MW, Mucha A, Lovell MR. Which on-field signs/symptoms predict protracted recovery from sport-related concussion among high school football players? Am J Sports Med. 2011;39:2311–8.

Chapter 4
Physical Examination

Carrie A. Jaworski and Stessie Zimmerman

Case

A 15-year-old female soccer player is on your ambulatory clinic schedule due to concern that she has sustained a sports-related concussion during a soccer game 3 days ago. The medical student rotating with you asks what tests and evaluations they should perform when they see this patient.

Patients with sports-related concussions often present to the primary care office for their initial evaluation. It is imperative for practitioners to conduct a focused and informed physical examination to guide further testing and recommended treatments. It is also essential that a practitioner pays special attention to the areas of the physical examination that lend themselves to an intervention that can augment the recovery of a patient with a concussion.

Research continues to be a priority to validate components of the physical examination for the evaluations of sports-related concussions. In addition, tools and applications are constantly being developed and advertised to clinicians for use in concussion evaluations that lack robust evidence to support their use. Recent publications stress the importance of developing a more standardized approach to examining a concussed patient to improve the quality of concussion research and ultimately improve patient outcomes.

At present, principal areas of the exam with support in the literature include mental status testing, cervical spine evaluation, balance testing, vestibulo-ocular examination, and orthostatic testing for select patients [1, 2]. The inclusion of

C. A. Jaworski (✉)
Intermountain Health, Park City, UT, USA
e-mail: CarrieA.Jaworski@imail.org

S. Zimmerman
Intermountain Health, Salt Lake City, UT, USA
e-mail: Stessie.Zimmerman@imail.org

© The Author(s), under exclusive license to Springer Nature Switzerland AG 2025
D. S. Patel (ed.), *Concussion Management for Primary Care*, https://doi.org/10.1007/978-3-031-85516-0_4

extremity and axial manual muscle strength evaluation, cranial nerve (CN) interrogation, and reflex testing is not specific for concussion. However, these tests are important to evaluate the other etiologies in the differential of a concussion [1]. Thus, these tests should be performed in the first evaluation and during subsequent evaluations if concern persists. In this chapter, each of these components of the physical exam will be explained with reference to available research supporting their use and an approach to the overall examination will be provided.

Question: Why are vital signs relevant in patients with concussions?

Changes in vital signs may be a helpful indicator in establishing the diagnosis of a concussion as well as when evaluating patients with persistent symptoms following a concussion. Head injuries are known to be associated with a temporary disruption of the autonomic system which can affect one's vital signs and cause symptoms both with changes in position and with activity [1]. This can be elicited by performing orthostatic vital signs (OVS). Orthostatic hypotension refers to a 20-mmHg or greater drop in systolic BP (SBP), a 10-mmHg or greater drop in diastolic BP (DBP), or a 30 beats per minute (bpm) increase in pulse from supine to standing positions with associated signs and symptoms of hypoperfusion [3]. The recommended way to evaluate OVS is with the orthostatic stress test (OST). A patient will have their BP and heart rate (HR) assessed after lying supine for 5 min, and then they will have BP and HR reassessed while standing at 1-, 3-, and 5-min intervals. Symptomatic changes are not necessary to make this diagnosis [3]. Of note, substitution of the seated for supine position can miss orthostatic hypotension in two-thirds of cases [4]. An increase in the heart rate may indicate signs of hypovolemia rather than autonomic dysfunction alone, which could point to an alternate etiology rather than being solely neurologic in nature [5]. Postural orthostatic tachycardia syndrome (POTS) and post-traumatic orthostatic tachycardia (OT) are other manifestations of autonomic dysregulation in which the HR increases without an associated drop in BP. POTS and OT are both defined as a sustained increase in HR $\geq$ 30 beats per minute (bpm) in patients older than 19 years and $\geq$ 40 bpm for patients $\leq$ 19 years of age in the absence of orthostatic hypotension after transitioning from supine to upright or with an upright tilt on the head-up tilt table test (HUT). Many concussion patients will have temporary signs and/or symptoms of orthostatic intolerance (OI) but will fail to meet the above diagnostic criteria for either POTS or OT [5]. Clinicians should monitor OVS for improvement in the patient with OI as it should improve as the patient's other concussion symptoms resolve. POTS and OT patients can often have similar presentations to a patient with persistent post-concussion symptoms (PPCS) requiring thoughtful consideration.

The Defense Centers of Excellence of Psychological Health and Traumatic Brain Injury recommends that patients with head injuries should be evaluated with OVS, especially when presenting with symptoms of dizziness [6]. OVS has good specificity of 75–90%, but sensitivity can be as low as 21%. HUT testing can be considered as an alternative test in the setting of a negative OVS where one still strongly suspects an autonomic component to the patient's symptoms [7]. HUT is not typically a first line approach in the evaluation of concussion, but it is often used in more recalcitrant cases or when overlap between conditions exists.

Autonomic dysregulation following a concussion has commonly been associated with exercise intolerance that provokes an increase in symptoms [8] in addition to contributing to impaired vestibular function that leads to problems with dizziness and coordination [9]. In the case of exercise intolerance, submaximal exercise testing can be performed on a bike or treadmill to evaluate a patient for their heart rate (HR) and blood pressure (BP) response to exercise [8]. One of the most recognized, and studied, protocols is known as the Buffalo Concussion Treadmill Test [8]. Performing these tests as part of the physical examination can inform rehabilitation recommendations [8]. The recovery of the autonomic nervous system following a concussion is vital for a patient to be able to tolerate exercise [8]. If the patient still complains of symptoms outside of exercise, one must continue the search for other contributing factors.

Question: How is a patient's mood and cognitive function impacted by a concussion?

Mental status changes in concussion can affect cognitive abilities, memory, and concentration in addition to emotional affect and lability. Currently available tools, such as the Standardized Assessment of Concussion [SAC] [10] and Sport Concussion Assessment Tool [SCAT] [2], offer a standardized assessment of the symptomology related to one's cognitive abilities. The SAC tool allows for immediate sideline mental status assessment of an athlete suspected of having a concussion. It assesses orientation, immediate memory, concentration, and delayed memory as well as includes an exertion test and a brief neurologic exam. It can be administered in approximately 5 minutes. Review of the literature suggests that, when used alone, the SAC does not reach statistical significance, but most experts still recommend its use as part of a more comprehensive evaluation of concussion [11]. According to the 6th International Conference on Concussion in Sport, the SCAT6 and Child SCAT6 (used for 8–12-year-olds) are intended to be used in the acute phase (< 7 days since injury). In contrast, the Sport Concussion Office Assessment Tool [SCOAT] SCOAT6 and Child SCOAT6 are new tools that are recommended for the office evaluation of patients with concern for concussion 7 or more days after injury [2]. These tools build upon other previous iterations including the SCAT, SCAT2, and SCAT5. There are many similarities between these prior versions of the test that have been validated [12], and edits to the SCAT6 result from expert consensus supporting its current use.

Changes in emotional state, particularly depressive symptoms, can severely impact quality of life for months after the injury [13]. Those who have a history of behavioral or mental illness, including post-traumatic stress disorder, affective disorders, substance use disorders, or attention deficit hyperactivity disorders, tend to have a higher risk of developing PPCS and prolonged mood instability [14, 15]. The Patient Health Questionnaire-9 (PHQ-9) is a validated depression screening tool that can serve as a useful adjunct to concussion screening when there is a high suspicion of a depression or affective disorder exacerbated or provoked by a concussion. The PHQ-9 is self-administered and can be used in multiple settings and populations [16, 17], examples including both concussed military personnel [18] and adolescents with traumatic brain injury (TBI) [19]. Additionally, the General Anxiety Disorder-7 (GAD-7) assessment tool can benefit clinicians in screening for anxiety disorders in patients following a concussion [20].

Question: What cranial nerve changes can be observed in patients following a concussion?

It is possible for one or more cranial nerves to sustain injuries even with minor head trauma, and these injuries may be missed if one is not astute during the physical exam [21, 22]. One study showed that 12.6% of patients with head trauma, including a significant number with mild TBI, had cranial nerve (CN) injuries [22]. In this study, CN II, CN III, and CN VII were the nerves most commonly injured [22]. In patients with mild TBI, CN I was most often found to be impaired with CNs II, IV, and VII being frequently injured as well [21]. In those with CN injuries, more than 80% showed abnormalities on head computed tomography scans [21]. This research suggests that physical examination of these nerves is particularly important to evaluate, whereas CN V and CNs IX–XII may be less revealing [21, 22]. Interestingly, up to 30% of patients diagnosed with a concussion experience anosmia or dyssomnia and CN I has a higher likelihood of injury in mild cases [21, 23]. That being said, CN I testing is frequently excluded from cranial nerve testing on most exams based on perceived difficulty with administration. An easy way to test is to keep coffee grounds in a sealed bag in exam rooms. It is unclear how injury to this nerve may affect appetite or nausea, but testing should be considered in concussion patients presenting with persistent anorexia or nausea. Table 4.1 outlines the approach to cranial nerve testing.

Question: What is the utility of evaluating vestibulo-ocular dysfunction, and what tests are most relevant for patients with concern for concussion?

Vestibular dysfunction is a common presenting sign seen with concussions and includes symptoms such as dizziness, vertigo, and difficulty with balance. Vestibular ocular dysfunction (VOD) is present in up to 76% of patients following mTBI in pediatric patients and in 50–90% of adult patients with concussions [24, 25]. Additionally, VOD can adversely affect one's quality of life with prolonged symptoms, higher risk of PPCS, and increased risk of disability [26, 27]. The differential remains large for concussed individuals who have dizziness and disequilibrium. One manifestation of disequilibrium following concussion is known as posttraumatic benign paroxysmal positional vertigo (BPPV). Following a concussion, adults demonstrate BPPV in 5–57% of cases. BPPV occurs less frequently in children and adolescence following concussion, reportedly in 5–20% of cases [28, 29]. Once VOD is diagnosed, it can be successfully treated with a rehabilitation program. Therefore, providers need to assess for this in their concussion evaluations and refer to rehabilitation specialists trained in concussion and comorbid vestibular and ocular disorders [30–33].

Table 4.1 Cranial nerve exam findings

Cranial nerve	Exam testing
CN I: olfactory nerve	Sense of smell with standardized order
CN II: optic nerve	Visual acuity Pupillary light reflex Visual fields
CN III: oculomotor nerve	Medial, superior, and inferior abduction movement of eye Accommodation of eyes
CN IV: trochlear nerve	Inferior adduction movement of eye
CN V: trigeminal nerve	Sensation of face Clamping of jaw
CN VI: abducens nerve	Lateral movement of eyes
CN VII: facial nerve	Facial movements (raise eyebrows, puff out cheeks, smile showing teeth) Taste of anterior 2/3 of tongue
CN VIII: vestibulocochlear nerve	Whispered hearing Assess for nystagmus
CN IX: glossopharyngeal nerve	Swallowing and pharyngeal gag reflex Taste of posterior 1/3 of tongue
CN X: vagus nerve	Gag reflex Visualization of uvula and posterior pharynx with phonation
CN XI: spinal accessory nerve	Manual muscle testing of sternocleidomastoid and trapezius
CN XII: hypoglossal nerve	Assess for tongue deviation with protrusion

Bolded nerves: most associated with concussions [21]

An ocular assessment with a focus on extraocular movements has become viewed as an increasingly important diagnostic tool used for concussions. Up to 40% of patients with TBIs exhibit ocular dysfunction such as impaired near point convergence, poor accommodation, and difficulties with oculomotor tracking [34, 35]. These vision problems often complicate return to school due to increased straining with computer use and reading [36]. The impairment of their function rises from shearing forces that injure the fiber tracts that connect the frontal cortex with the cerebellum. This can cause difficulty with coordination of eye traction on a fixed point which can worsen with increased mental tasks [37].

Vestibular/Ocular Motor Screening

Vestibular/ocular motor screening (VOMS) has become a well-accepted method of evaluating a concussion patient's vestibulo-ocular system. The assessment includes five domains: [1] smooth pursuits, [2] horizontal and vertical saccades, [8] near point of convergence (NPC), [9] horizontal vestibulo-ocular reflex (VOR), and [3] visual motion sensitivity (VMS). A cross-sectional study of the VOMS assessment tool reflected good internal consistency and proved to be a reliable method of identifying patients with a concussion. New research suggests that the use of modified

VOMS testing which consists of smooth pursuits, horizontal saccades, horizontal VOR, and VMS resulted in equivalent identification of vestibulo-ocular deficits in concussion patients [38, 39]. See demonstration of VOMS testing.

Saccades and Smooth Pursuits

Both saccades and smooth pursuit testing have demonstrated high sensitivity and specificity in helping to determine prognosis in recovering from concussions [40]. Abnormal extraocular tests have been associated with worse outcomes and have been more predictive for the development of PPCS than neuropsychological testing, arm motor function, or patient self-report of symptoms [40]. Furthermore, patients diagnosed with PPCS had worse visual tracking when compared with controls [40, 41].

Nystagmus

Nystagmus is a common finding in children who have sustained head trauma. Up to 46% of children may have spontaneous and/or positional nystagmus after head trauma and 20% will continue to demonstrate abnormal findings for 6–12 months after injury [42]. Vertical or asymmetric nystagmus after a head injury may signify a more pathologic issue such as a brainstem lesion and should prompt emergent imaging and/or referral [43].

Accommodation and Convergence

Normal near point of convergence (NPC) ranges from 6 to 10 cm. Individuals who have sustained a concussion often develop spasm or dysfunction of the ocular muscles responsible for near point convergence [44]. This can lead a concussed patient to have double vision when focusing on an object that is greater than 6–10 cm away. Age-related changes in the eye result in lower values for normal NPC in children than in adults. NPC can be obtained quantitatively using a standard accommodation ruler. Convergence insufficiency has been known to affect reading speed and comprehension [45]. This is especially problematic for adolescents and can delay their readiness for return to the classroom. Isolated convergence insufficiency has been shown to be responsible for visual symptoms in 9% of individuals who have sustained a TBI [46]. One study showed that 69% of adolescents with a concussion had one or more vision abnormalities: 51% had accommodative disorders, 49% had convergence insufficiency, and 29% had saccadic dysfunction [47].

King-Devick

The King-Devick test is a test that has been utilized to track eye movements and is advertised heavily since it can be administered by a lay person such as a teacher or parent at a very low to no cost [48]. It has demonstrated benefit in the acute evaluation of a concussion 0–6 hours and 24–48 hours following injury with 80% sensitivity but has poor specificity at 46% and 41% at these respective time points [49]. However, this test is not necessary for a concussion evaluation in the office setting.

Fundoscopy

A fundoscopic evaluation is a known valuable tool to assess for papilledema due to increased intracranial pressure after head trauma. However, it is low yield in the setting of concussions since papilledema occurs in only 3.5% of severe head trauma cases [50]. It is also very operator-dependent and relies on the experience of the physician to accurately identify signs of papilledema [51, 52]. Nonetheless, clinicians should use their best judgment in terms of utilization of this test.

Question: Is balance testing useful in the evaluation of a concussion?

Concussions are associated with abnormalities in balance and equilibrium both in static and dynamic testing [53]. The Balance Error Scoring System (BESS) is frequently used in assessing athletes who have sustained concussions [54], but, despite this, there are several noted drawbacks including length of time of testing which can take 5–7 min, low sensitivity [55], limited reliability between multiple tests [56], and high false-positive rates [57]. Additionally, sensitivity for diagnosing concussion drops days following concussions as balance appears to normalize over the first 3–5 days [58].

The Romberg test, though frequently administered in clinical office settings, also has low yield for assessing vestibular dysfunction [59]. On the other hand, tandem gait and coordination tests, such as finger-to-nose tests, have been found to have good reliability when used in the assessment of concussions [60]. The complex tandem gait evaluation includes the evaluation of balance in four stations: tandem gait with eyes open going forward, eyes closed going forward, eyes open going backward, and eyes closed going backward. The evaluator measures errors or sway during the patient's performance of this gait. Complex tandem gait testing is predictive of PPCS in pediatric patients as well [61].

Question: Why is it important to assess the cervical spine (C-spine) in a concussion exam?

When assessing head injuries, it is essential to evaluate for any signs of neck injury as the two can closely imitate each other and coexist. Among sports-related patients with concussions up to 43% report neck pain [62]. Cervical muscle strain caused by whiplash injuries may present with headaches, dizziness, disequilibrium, visual changes, and poor balance similar to that of concussions [63–65]. It is important to palpate the C-spine and, if negative, also apply resisted cervical isometric forces at the higher cervical levels. If pain is reproduced with these maneuvers, this should prompt cervical spine X-rays with flexion and extension views and potentially advanced imaging [63]. The Spurling test is useful in determining signs of cervical nerve root irritation, which can be due to a herniated disc or possible dislocation. It is performed by extending and rotating the patient's head toward the arm on the side being tested and applying an axial force to the head. A positive test results if the patient develops shooting pain down the arm with this maneuver [1].

Cervical proprioception is another important physical exam test that provides spatial orientation of how the head is positioned and moves relative to the trunk. It can be tested by having a patient close his or her eyes, rotate the neck, and try to bring his or her head and neck to a neutral position within 5 degrees [66]. It is useful to assess as it can be associated with symptoms of disequilibrium [66]. Abnormalities with cervical proprioception can be treated with specific proprioceptive rehabilitation and, if undetected, may lead to prolonged symptoms [64].

Additionally, it is important to assess for both temporomandibular joint dysfunction and thoracic abnormalities as these can also coexist with concussions and contribute to headache, tinnitus, dizziness, neck pain [67], thoracic winging [68], and thoracic myofascial trigger points [69].

Question: What additional neurologic evaluation should be considered in concussion testing?

There is not enough evidence to state whether manual muscle testing (MMT) or deep tendon reflexes (DTR) are affected by concussion. However, the rationale for testing muscle strength, DTRs, and the remainder of the neurologic examination is to exclude more serious pathology. Focal muscle weakness with absent or hypoactive reflexes may indicate a brainstem or cerebellar lesion [70]. On the other hand, findings such as hyperreflexia, finger rolling, pronator drift, Hoffman's sign, and a Babinski sign can signify an upper neuron injury of the cerebral cortex [70]. See Table 4.2 for further rationale of specific physical exam tests.

Question: How can the physical examination be adapted for evaluation of the para athlete with concern for concussion?

Much of the previous discussion assumes that a patient at baseline can see, hear, walk, comprehend, speak, have manual dexterity, and/or safely move the cervical spine. These assumptions may be incorrect and could put the patient at risk if these beliefs are maintained in the evaluation of the para athlete or the athlete with an intellectual disability. It is imperative whenever possible to obtain a baseline evaluation, particularly in these patients, to better identify relevant changes during an evaluation for a concussion. Novel techniques can be implemented to adapt the physical exam to meet the needs of the patient. For example, the wheelchair error scoring system could be used in lieu of the complex tandem gait in veteran wheelchair athletes [71]. The Concussion in Para Sport (CIPS) group published a first

Table 4.2 Rationale for physical exam tests in concussion

Physical exam test	Utility
Orthostatic vital signs	Recommended particularly for patients presenting with dizziness and lightheadedness Signifies autonomic dysregulation and can help distinguish other causes from a concussion Changes in heart rate is a relevant finding particularly in the pediatric population
Mental status	Refers to changes in cognition, memory, concentration, and mood SCAT6, child SCAT6, SCOAT6, and child SCOAT6 include sections to assess cognitive function Patients with prior histories of mental illness are at increased risk for persistent post-concussive symptoms
Cranial nerve exam	Important to rule out CN injuries when evaluating for concussions as they can often be missed CN I is most injured with a concussion while injuries in CN V and CNs IX–XII are less likely to occur
Vestibulo-ocular evaluation	Often presents with signs of dizziness, vertigo, and balance difficulty which can persist if untreated Dynamic visual acuity should be considered for testing of vestibulo-ocular dysfunction Ocular dysfunction presents with impaired near point convergence, accommodation, and oculomotor tracking and can significantly impact school and work function
Saccades and smooth pursuits	Highly sensitive and specific to help determine prognosis with concussions Abnormal tests associated with higher risk of persistent post-concussive symptoms
Nystagmus	Horizontal nystagmus is a common finding in patients with head trauma Vertical nystagmus may indicate a brainstem lesion and warrants urgent imaging
Accommodation and convergence	Normal near point convergence is 6–10 cm Ocular muscle dysfunction contributes to difficulties with convergence which can affect reading speed and comprehension Helpful in determining classroom readiness
Balance Assessment	Balance Error Score System (BESS) is frequently utilized despite limited reliability Romberg test is low-yield Complex tandem gait and coordination tests may be more meaningful findings in balance assessment of concussed patients, particularly in pediatric patients
Musculoskeletal exam	Focus on head and neck for trauma and range of motion Consider TMJ, and thoracic spine evaluation based on the history and mechanism of injury
Neurologic assessment	MMT and DTR evaluation is important to evaluate for other ominous neurologic diagnoses following a head or neck injury

position statement in 2021 to assist clinicians with their approach to evaluating the para athlete with a suspected concussion [72].

Key Points
- The diagnosis and evaluation of concussions are complicated by the fact that many symptoms overlap between concussions and other conditions.
- Utilizing physical exam techniques that correlate with the known physiologic processes disturbed by a concussive injury can improve the accuracy of the diagnosis of concussions.
- It is important to maximize the use of validated tools and examination methods to detect injury patterns and abnormalities.
- A standardized approach will allow multiple physicians involved to communicate more effectively and track patient findings more clearly over time. It can also help to detect patient abnormalities that would benefit from rehabilitation therapies thus aiding in a more expedient recovery. However, patient-specific factors, time, and resource limitations should also influence which parts of the evaluation are performed and by whom.
- Adaptations can be made to improve the utility of the physical examination when evaluating para athletes for sports-related concussions.
- A more evidence-based approach to the physical exam will lend itself to further research in this field and improve patient outcomes.

References

1. Haider MN, Leddy JJ, Du W, Macfarlane J. Practical management: brief physical examination for sport-related concussion in the outpatient setting. Clin J Sport Med. 2020;30(5):513–7. https://doi.org/10.1097/JSM.0000000000000687.
2. Patricios JS, Schneider KJ, Dvorak J, Ahmed OH, Blauwet C, et al. Consensus statement on concussion in sport: the 6th International Conference on Concussion in Sport-Amsterdam. Br J Sports Med. 2023;57(11):695–711. https://doi.org/10.1136/bjsports-2023-106898.
3. Consensus Committee of the American Autonomic Society and the American Academy of Neurology. Consensus statement on the definition of orthostatic hypotension, pure autonomic failure, and multiple system atrophy. Neurology. 1996;46(5):1470.
4. Cooke J, Carew S, O'Connor M, Costelloe A, Sheehy T, Lyons D. Sitting and standing blood pressure measurements are not accurate for the diagnosis of orthostatic hypotension. QJM. 2009;102:335–9.
5. Pearson R, Sheridan CA, Kang K, Brown A, Baham M, Asarnow R, Giza CC, Choe MC. Post-concussive orthostatic tachycardia is distinct from postural orthostatic tachycardia syndrome (POTS) in children and adolescents. Child Neurol Open. 2022;9:2329048X221082753. https://doi.org/10.1177/2329048X221082753.
6. Defense Centers of Excellence for Psychological Traumatic Brain Injury. Assessment and management of dizziness associated with mild TBI. 2012.: http://www.dcoe.health.mil/Content/Navigation/Documents/Dizziness_Associated_with_Mild_TBI_Clinical_Recommendation.pdf. Accessed 3 Oct 2019
7. Faraji F, Kinsella LJ, Rutledge JC, Mikulec AA. The comparative usefulness of orthostatic testing and tilt table testing in the evaluation of autonomic-associated dizziness. Otol Neurotol. 2011;32:654–9.

8. Leddy JJ, Haider MN, Ellis MJ, Mannix R, Darling SR, Freitas MS, Suffoletto HN, Leiter J, Cordingley DM, Willer B. Early Subthreshold aerobic exercise for sport-related concussion: a randomized clinical trial. JAMA Pediatr. 2019;173(4):319–25. https://doi.org/10.1001/jamapediatrics.2018.4397.
9. Kanjwal K, Karabin B, Kanjwal Y, Grubb BP. Autonomic dysfunction presenting as postural tachycardia syndrome following traumatic brain injury. Cardiol J. 2010;17:482–7.
10. McCrea M. Standardized mental status assessment of sports concussion. Clin J Sport Med. 2001;11:176–81.
11. Grubenhoff JA, Kirkwood M, Goa D, Deakyne S, Wathen J. Evaluation of the standardized assessment of concussion in a pediatric emergency department. Pediatrics. 2010;126(4):688–95.
12. Lumba-Brown A, Yeates KO, Sarmiento K, et al. Centers for disease control and prevention guideline on the diagnosis and management of mild traumatic brain injury among children. JAMA Pediatr. 2018;172(11)
13. Bombardier CH, Fann JR, Temkin NR, Esselman PC, Barber J, Dikmen SS. Rates of major depressive disorder and clinical outcomes following traumatic brain injury. JAMA. 2010;303:1938–45.
14. Evered L, Ruff R, Baldo J, Isomura A. Emotional risk factors and postconcussional disorder. Assessment. 2003;10:420–7.
15. Iverson GL. Misdiagnosis of the persistent postconcussion syndrome in patients with depression. Arch Clin Neuropsychol. 2006;21:303–10.
16. Richardson LP, McCauley E, Grossman DC, et al. Evaluation of the Patient Health Questionnaire–9 Item for detecting major depression among adolescents. Pediatrics. 2010;126:1117–23.
17. Silverberg ND, Bombardier C, Hallam B. Screening for depression after mild traumatic brain injury. http://www.ubcphysmed.org?LinkClick.aspx?fileticket=-FNZSEDPx7w%3D&tabid=109. Accessed October 12, 2019.
18. Rosenthal JF, Erickson JC. Post-traumatic stress disorder in U.S. soldiers with post-traumatic headache. Headache. 2013;53:1564–72.
19. O'Connor SS, Zatzick DF, Wang J, et al. Association between posttraumatic stress, depression, and functional impairments in adolescents 24 months after traumatic brain injury. J Trauma Stress. 2012;25:264–71.
20. Zachar-Tirado CN, Donders J. Clinical utility of the GAD-7 in identifying anxiety disorders after traumatic brain injury. Brain Inj. 2021;35(6):655–60. https://doi.org/10.1080/02699052.2021.1895315.
21. Coello AF, Canals AG, Gonzalez JM, Martin JJ. Cranial nerve injury after minor head trauma. J Neurosurg. 2010;113:547–55.
22. Patel P, Kalyanaraman S, Reginald J, et al. Post-traumatic cranial nerve injury. Indian J Neurotrauma. 2005;2:27–32.
23. Callahan CD, Hinkebein JH. Assessment of anosmia after traumatic brain injury: performance characteristics of the University of Pennsylvania smell identification test. J Head Trauma Rehabil. 2002;17:251–6.
24. Cicerone CM, Hoffman DD, Gowdy PD, Kim JS. The perception of color from motion. Percept Psychophys. 1995;57:761–77.
25. Kaae C, Cadigan K, Lai K, Theis J. Vestibulo-ocular dysfunction in mTBI: utility of the VOMS for evaluation and management – a review. NeuroRehabilitation. 2022;50(3):279–96. https://doi.org/10.3233/NRE-228012.
26. Gottshall KR, Hoffer ME. Tracking recovery of vestibular function in individuals with blast-induced head trauma using vestibular-visual-cognitive interaction tests. J Neurol Phys Ther. 2010;34:94–7.
27. Hoffer ME, Gottshall KR, Moore R, Balough BJ, Wester D. Characterizing and treating dizziness after mild head trauma. Otol Neurotol. 2004;25:135–8.

28. Bogle JM. Vestibular and balance dysfunction following sport-related concussion. Perspectives of the ASHA Special Interest Groups. 2019;4(6):1349–63. https://doi.org/10.1044/2019_PERS-SIG6-2019-0004.
29. Gottshall K. Vestibular rehabilitation after mild traumatic brain injury with vestibular pathology. Neuro Rehabilitation. 2011;29:167–71.
30. Alsalaheen BA, Mucha A, Morris LO, et al. Vestibular rehabilitation for dizziness and balance disorders after concussion. J Neurol Phys Ther. 2010;34:87–93.
31. Gottshall K, Drake A, Gray N, McDonald E, Hoffer ME. Objective vestibular tests as outcome measures in head injury patients. Laryngoscope. 2003;113:1746–50.
32. Liu H. Presentation and outcome of post-traumatic benign paroxysmal positional vertigo. Acta Otolaryngol. 2012;132:803–6.
33. Burgio DL, Blakley BW, Myers SF. The high-frequency oscillopsia test. J Vestib Res. 1992;2:221–6.
34. Green W, Ciuffreda KJ, Thiagarajan P, Szymanowicz D, Ludlam DP, Kapoor N. Static and dynamic aspects of accommodation in mild traumatic brain injury: a review. Optometry. 2010;81:129–36.
35. Szymanowicz D, Ciuffreda KJ, Thiagarajan P, Ludlam DP, Green W, Kapoor N. Vergence in mild traumatic brain injury: a pilot study. J Rehabil Res Dev. 2012;49:1083–100.
36. Halstead ME, McAvoy K, Devore CD, et al. Returning to learning following a concussion. Pediatrics. 2013;132:948–57.
37. Contreras R, Ghajar J, Bahar S, Suh M. Effect of cognitive load on eye-target synchronization during smooth pursuit eye movement. Brain Res. 2011;1398:55–63.
38. Ferris LM, Konots AP, Eagle SR, Elbin RJ, Clugston JR, Ortega J, Port NL. Optimizing VOMS for identifying acute concussion in collegiate athletes: findings from the NCAA-DoD CARE consortium. Vision Res. 2022;200:108081.
39. Mucha A, Collins MW, Elbin RJ, et al. A brief vestibular/ocular motor screening (VOMS) assessment to evaluate concussions: preliminary findings. Am J Sports Med. 2014;42:2479–86.
40. Heitger MH, Jones RD, Anderson TJ. A new approach to predicting postconcussion syndrome after mild traumatic brain injury based upon eye movement function. Conf Proc IEEE Eng Med Biol Soc. 2008;2008:3570–3.
41. Heitger MH, Jones RD, Macleod AD, Snell DL, Frampton CM, Anderson TJ. Impaired eye movements in post-concussion syndrome indicate suboptimal brain function beyond the influence of depression, malingering or intellectual ability. Brain. 2009;132(pt 10):2850–70.
42. Vartiainen E, Karjalainen S, Karja J. Vestibular disorders following head injury in children. Int J Pediatr Otorhinolaryngol. 1985;9:135–41.
43. Shawkat FS, Kriss A, Thompson D, Russell-Eggitt I, Taylor D, Harris C. Vertical or asymmetric nystagmus need not imply neurological disease. Br J Ophthalmol. 2000;84:175–80.
44. Scheiman M, Gallaway M, Frantz KA, et al. Nearpoint of convergence: test procedure, target selection, and normative data. Optom Vis Sci. 2003;80:214–25.
45. Thiagarajan P, Ciuffreda KJ, Ludlam DP. Vergence dysfunction in mild traumatic brain injury (mTBI): a review. Ophthalmic Physiol Opt. 2011;31:456–68.
46. Alvarez TL, Kim EH, Vicci VR, Dhar SK, Biswal BB, Barrett AM. Concurrent vision dysfunctions in convergence insufficiency with traumatic brain injury. Optom Vis Sci. 2012;89:1740–51.
47. Master CL, Scheiman M, Gallaway M, et al. Vision diagnoses are common after concussion in adolescents. Clin Pediatr (Phila). 2016;55:260–7.
48. Leong DF, Balcer LJ, Galetta SL, Liu Z, Master CL. The King-Devick test as a concussion screening tool administered by sports parents. J Sports Med Phys Fitness. 2014;54:70–7.
49. Le RK, Ortega J, Chrisman SP, Kontos AP, Buckley TA, Kaminski TW, Meyer BP, Clugston JR, Goldman JT, McAllister T, McCrea M, Broglio SP, Schmidt JD. King-Devick sensitivity and specificity to concussion in collegiate athletes. J Athl Train. 2023;58(2):97–105. https://doi.org/10.4085/1062-6050-0063.21.

50. Selhorst JB, Gudeman SK, Butterworth JF 4th, Harbison JW, Miller JD, Becker DP. Papilledema after acute head injury. Neurosurgery. 1985;16:357–63.
51. Steffen H, Eifert B, Aschoff A, Kolling GH, Volcker HE. The diagnostic value of optic disc evaluation in acute elevated intracranial pressure. Ophthalmology. 1996;103:1229–32.
52. Johnson LN, Hepler RS, Bartholomew MJ. Accuracy of papilledema and pseudopapilledema detection: a multispecialty study. J Fam Pract. 1991;33:381–6.
53. Harmon KG, Drezner J, Gammons M, et al. American medical society for sports medicine position statement: concussion in sport. Clin J Sport Med. 2013;23:1–18.
54. Davis GA, Iverson GL, Guskiewicz KM, Ptito A, Johnston KM. Contributions of neuroimaging, balance testing, electrophysiology and blood markers to the assessment of sport-related concussion. Br J Sports Med. 2009;43(suppl 1):i36–45.
55. McCrea M, Barr WB, Guskiewicz K, et al. Standard regression-based methods for measuring recovery after sport-related concussion. J Int Neuropsychol Soc. 2005;11:58–69.
56. Finnoff JT, Peterson VJ, Hollman JH, Smith J. Intrarater and interrater reliability of the Balance Error Scoring System (BESS). PM R. 2009;1:50–4.
57. Mulligan I, Boland M, Payette J. Prevalence of neurocognitive and balance deficits in collegiate aged football players without clinically diagnosed concussion. J Orthop Sports Phys Ther. 2012;42:625–32.
58. Bell DR, Guskiewicz KM, Clark MA, Padua DA. Systematic review of the balance error scoring system. Sports Health. 2011;3:287–95.
59. Jacobson GP, McCaslin DL, Piker EG, Gruenwald J, Grantham S, Tegel L. Insensitivity of the "Romberg test of standing balance on firm and compliant support surfaces" to the results of caloric and VEMP tests. Ear Hear. 2011;32:e1–5.
60. Schneiders AG, Sullivan SJ, Gray AR, Hammond-Tooke GD, McCrory PR. Normative values for three clinical measures of motor performance used in the neurological assessment of sports concussion. J Sci Med Sport. 2010;13:196–201.
61. Maser CL, Master SR, Wiebe DJ, et al. Vision and vestibular system dysfunction predicts prolonged concussion recovery in children. Clin J Sport Med. 2018;28:139–45.
62. Oyekan AA, Eagle S, Trbovich AM, Shaw JD, Schneider M, Collins M, Lee JY, Kontos AP. Neck symptoms and associated clinical outcomes in patients following concussion. J Head Trauma Rehabil. 2023;38(6):417–24. https://doi.org/10.1097/HTR.0000000000000866.
63. Crutchfield K, Rivenburgh D, Morris L, Werner J. Atlanto-axial subluxation: treatable cause of post concussion syndrome. Neurology. 2014;82(suppl):P5.305.
64. Leddy JJ, Baker JG, Merchant A, et al. Brain or strain? Symptoms alone do not distinguish physiologic concussion from cervical/vestibular injury. Clin J Sport Med. 2015;25:237–42.
65. Treleaven J. Dizziness, unsteadiness, visual disturbances, and postural control: implications for the transition to chronic symptoms after a whiplash trauma. Spine. 2011;36(suppl):S211–7.
66. Armstrong B, McNair P, Taylor D. Head and neck position sense. Sports Med. 2008;38:101–17.
67. Packard RC. Epidemiology and pathogenesis of posttraumatic headache. J Head Trauma Rehabil. 1999;14:9–21.
68. Martin RM, Fish DE. Scapular winging: anatomical review, diagnosis, and treatments. Curr Rev Musculoskel Med. 2008;1:1–11.
69. Page P. Cervicogenic headaches: an evidence-led approach to clinical management. Int J Sports Phys Ther. 2011;6:254–66.
70. Anderson NE, Mason DF, Fink JN, Bcrgin PS, Charleston AJ, Gamble GD. Detection of focal cerebral hemisphere lesions using the neurological examination. J Neurol Neurosurg Psychiatry. 2005;76:545–9.
71. Harper MW, Lee J, Sherman KA, Uihlein MJ, Lee KKK. Wheelchair athlete concussion baseline data: a pilot retrospective analysis. Am J Phys Med Rehabil. 2021;100(9):895–9. https://doi.org/10.1097/PHM.0000000000001630.
72. Weiler R, Blauwet C, Clarke D, et al. Concussion in para sport: the first position statement of the Concussion in Para Sport (CIPS) Group. Br J Sports Med. 2021;55:1187–95.

Chapter 5
Diagnostic Tests for Concussion

Alan Shahtaji, Sam Galloway, and Michelle Doscas

Clinical Case

A 17-year-old female is brought into your outpatient primary care clinic after being elbowed in the head last night while challenging for a header in her soccer match. Her parents want to know what is the best diagnostic test to confirm a concussion?

There is no single best test to diagnose a concussion. Rather, the diagnosis of acute concussion requires a multifaceted approach that takes into account the history surrounding the injury, signs and symptoms at that time, as well as subsequent signs and symptoms upon evaluation in the clinic. The tools described below are part of this initial evaluation and can be implemented in the clinic to help aid the primary care physician in making a diagnosis of concussion.

Table 5.1 (below) summarizes the diagnostic utility of the tests discussed in this chapter.

Post-concussion Symptom Scale (Checklist)

Question: If someone completes a symptom checklist without any symptoms does that rule out a concussion?

A. Shahtaji (✉) · S. Galloway
Department of Family Medicine, Division of Sports Medicine,
University of California at San Diego, San Diego, CA, USA
e-mail: ashahtaji@health.ucsd.edu

M. Doscas
Silicon Valley Sports Medicine, Campbell, CA, USA

© The Author(s), under exclusive license to Springer Nature
Switzerland AG 2025
D. S. Patel (ed.), *Concussion Management for Primary Care*,
https://doi.org/10.1007/978-3-031-85516-0_5

Table 5.1 Diagnostic concussion testing summary

Diagnostic tests	Pros	Cons
PCSS	Best used in first 7 days May help predict recovery timeline Low cost [1, 2]	Subjective report that requires patient honesty [1, 2]
SAC	Best used in first 48 h [2] Objective cognitive test Can be done on the sideline Low-cost [3]	Limited in return to play decision-making [3]
BESS/mBESS	Best used in first 7 days [2] Good assessment of postural stability	BESS requires foam pad, which may not be available in an office setting If baseline testing is done, post-injury testing should be completed by the same provider [2]
SCAT6	Most reliable in first 3 days, can be used up to 7 days after injury Can be completed in 10–15 mins PCSS, SAC, and mBESS are embedded in the SCAT6 [4]	Limited in tracking recovery and return to play [4]
MACE2	Used for military concussion assessment [5]	Limited use >12–24 h post-injury [5]
K-D test	Takes 2 minutes to complete Can be done on the sideline [6–8]	Debated validity in recent literature [9] Fee to use [6]
VOMS	High internal consistency, relatively low false-positive rate [10]	Not validated for sideline use [10]
Eye tracking	Does not require baseline test Good test-retest reliability [11, 12]	Expensive technology [11, 12]
Force plate/ BTrackS	Objective Eliminates inter-observer variability [13]	Expensive Requires high-tech equipment [13]
Orthostatic vital signs	Easy to use in clinic [14]	Limited data re: predictive capacity [14]
Buffalo Concussion Treadmill Test	Helpful for diagnosis, prognosis, and developing patient-specific exercise recommendations [15]	Limited access in primary care clinic [15]

The Post-Concussion Symptom Scale (PCSS) is a list of symptoms separated into four categories: physical, emotional, cognitive, and sleep. The athlete is asked to grade the severity of these symptoms on a scale of 0 (absent) to 6 (most severe).

One study noted a 97.5% sensitivity of the PCSS alone when used within 24 h post-injury in collegiate athletes [1, 2]. In 24–48 h after injury, 100% of patients reported elevated symptoms on the PCSS [2]. On day 3, 97%; day 4, 93%; day 5, 76%; and day 7, 64%, of athletes reported elevated symptoms, respectively. Cognitive and physical symptom scores are typically the highest immediately after concussion [2]. This test can be particularly useful as recent research suggests that symptom burden may help prognosticate duration of recovery [16, 17]. Nevertheless, the subjective nature of this test is dependent on the athlete's honesty and ability to correctly identify their symptoms. For this reason, the PCSS *alone* is not useful in diagnosing a concussion. Adolescents with preexisting conditions such as ADHD, mental health diagnoses, learning disabilities, headaches/migraines, or prior concussions may score higher on this test [18]. Having baseline preseason testing may be helpful in this subgroup. It is important to use the symptom scale in conjunction with an appropriate physical exam and additional screening tools to assess for concussion.

Standardized Assessment of Concussion (SAC)

Question: Is the Standardized Assessment of Concussion (SAC) more objective than the symptom checklist?

The Standardized Assessment of Concussion (SAC) is a 5- to 10-min written test with a total composite score of 30 points that includes four domains of cognitive function: orientation, immediate recall, concentration, and delayed recall [3]. This test has demonstrated its usefulness in ease of administration as well as its ability to detect subtle differences in mental status changes. The greatest differences in mean scores can be seen within the first 48 h after injury [2]. Similarly, large effects were appreciated when the SAC was conducted directly after the injury. Unlike the PCSS, this test gathers objective data and therefore is not dependent on the subjective report from the injured athlete. This test can be used as an initial tool to help in diagnosis, as well as to track patients' recovery over time. It is limited in its ability to guide return to play/learn decisions, however, as research has suggested that 50% of injured athletes still had symptoms at the time that their SAC score returned to baseline with some studies reporting it to be as soon as 2 days after injury [19, 20].

BESS/mBESS: Balance Error Scoring System

Question: What are the pros and cons of using the mBESS over the BESS?

The Balance Error Scoring System (BESS) is a low-cost approach in evaluating static postural stability for an athlete with a suspected concussion and can be done in any exam room. (See the Physical Examination of Concussion Chapter for further details.) The exam takes up to 10 min to conduct and requires two different testing surfaces: a firm surface such as the ground and a 2.5-inch thick foam surface. The patient performs three different stances to be held 20 seconds at a time: the double-leg stance, single-leg stance, and tandem stance initially on a firm surface and then on a foam surface. Every error made (refer to Fig. 5.1) equals one point, so a higher score indicates more postural instability.

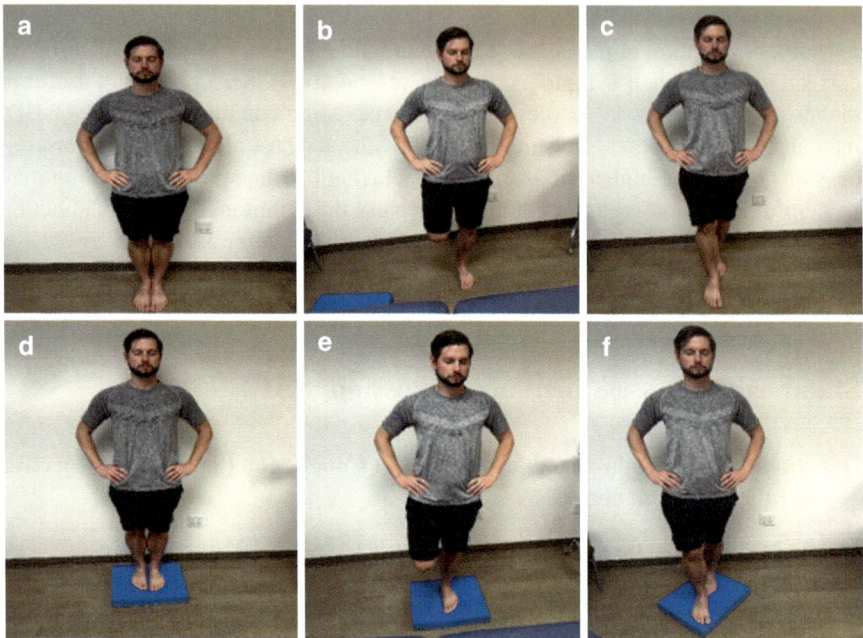

Double Leg Stance   Single leg stance   Tandem stance

Errors: Lifting hands off of the iliac crests • Opening eyes • Stepping, stumbling, or falling • Flexing or abducting hip more than 30° • Lifting the forefoot or heel • Remaining out of the testing position for more than 5 s

Fig. 5.1 Balance error scoring system

The BESS has a sensitivity of 60% within the first 7 days after injury [2]. The use of pre-injury baseline balance testing for all athletes has insufficient evidence to support its practice [2]. If pre-injury baseline testing is done, it is important to note that there is a higher inter-rater minimum detectable change score compared with intra-rater, which indicates the importance of the same provider completing the baseline BESS and post-injury BESS if possible [2].

The modified Balance Error Scoring System (mBESS) eliminates the foam pad and is therefore more practical in the primary care setting. Compared with the BESS, the mBESS has a higher sensitivity (71%) within 7 days post-injury [2]. The inter-rater reliability of the mBESS is noted to be fair to strong [2]. The mBESS is embedded in the SCAT 6.

It is important to note that often the tests discussed so far in this chapter are used in combination to help diagnose an acute concussion. One study noted a combination of a symptom score (PCSS), SAC, and mBESS resulted in sensitivities of 61% within 1 hour post-injury, 67% 1–24 h post-injury and 55% 24–72 h post-injury [2].

SCAT6

Question: Is there a cutoff score on the SCAT6 that can be used to reliably diagnose concussion?
Sport Concussion Assessment Tool 6 (SCAT6) (bmj.com)

The Sport Concussion Assessment Tool (SCAT) is arguably the most widely used standardized method of evaluating those with a suspected concussion in patients aged 13 years and older. It has undergone numerous revisions to include a more comprehensive evaluation, with the most current 6th edition (SCAT6) released in 2023. It is a written test that can be implemented in the clinic, requiring 10–15 mins to conduct, and can be compared with a preseason/baseline SCAT6 assessment (although this is not required). It includes an emergency/on-field and off-field assessment, but for the purposes of this chapter, we will focus on the latter.

The off-field assessment implements these commonly used diagnostic tools [4]:

1. Patient demographics (focusing on history of head injuries and neuro/psychological diagnoses)
2. Symptom evaluation (PCSS)
3. Cognitive screening using SAC (with added timed component for months in reverse)
4. Coordination/balance screening, including mBESS (with new timed tandem gait)
5. Delayed recall (expanded to ten-word recall)
6. Decision documentation for the provider

There are also optional components of the SCAT6 [4]:

1. Using a foam pad for the balance testing
2. Dual task tandem gait, which includes the timed tandem gait while also having the patient count backward by 7s

The SCAT has high diagnostic utility that is generalizable to the larger population with only low to moderate levels of bias and is most reliable in the first 3 days post-injury but can be used up to 7 days post-injury [4]. As a result, the SCAT is more valuable in helping to make the initial diagnosis of concussion rather than tracking recovery and assisting return to play/learn decision-making [2]. Compared to prior versions, the SCAT6 adds a ten-word recall and timed sections to the cognitive component. This decision was made due to a ceiling effect noted with the prior five-word recall [2]. There is also a revised coordination/balance section to include a dual-task tandem gait, which asks the patient to perform a timed tandem gait while also completing a cognitive task such as backward serial 7s. In one study, this test alone had 84.8% sensitivity and 72.4% specificity [21]. However, more research is needed to further evaluate whether these changes help improve diagnostic utility in the acute and subacute post-injury evaluations.

While the cervical spine exam is not included in the off-field/initial office assessment, it is the recommendation of the chapter authors to include this in the physical examination.

Child SCAT6

Question: Is there an alternative to SCAT6 for younger children?
Child SCAT6

The child SCAT6 is meant for use in children from 8 to 12 years old and is consistent in format with the traditional SCAT6 [22]. To yield the highest accuracy, the test should be conducted in no less than 10–15 min. Major differences compared with the traditional SCAT6 are omission of orientation questions, modification of the symptom scale, and addition of parent observation of symptoms [22]. The child SCAT6 has added timed cognitive testing, more complex balance testing, and updated return to learn and sport protocols [23]. Within the Child SCAT6, the child and parent symptom scale has the highest internal consistency and stability over time [2]. As with the traditional SCAT6, a limitation is the lack of data available in regard to its validity for patients with learning disabilities and across different cultures and languages [24].

Military Acute Concussion Evaluation 2 (MACE 2)

Question: How does MACE 2 compare to SAC when evaluating athletes more than 24–48 h after injury?
https://www.health.mil/Reference-Center/Publications/2020/07/30/Military-Acute-Concussion-Evaluation-MACE-2

The Military Acute Concussion Evaluation 2 (MACE 2) was revised in 2021 and is designed to assess the likelihood of a concussion for patients in a military operational setting. The MACE 2 was updated to include an expanded history and red flag section as well as a more detailed vestibular ocular motor screening (VOMS) [5]. The Standardized Assessment of Concussion (SAC), discussed above, is embedded within the MACE 2 [5]. The MACE 2 is made up of a total of 30 points with the mean non-concussed patient scoring 27 and a score of 25 or less indicative of an acute concussion versus other, more serious brain injury (sensitivity 11–40%, specificity 80–96%) [25]. Similar to the SAC, the MACE 2 was designed to be administered acutely as it demonstrated declining sensitivity/specificity when administered more than 12–24 h after the event. Military personnel have expressed confidence in their ability to use this tool effectively [26]. Furthermore, as with other diagnostic tests, there is no cutoff value that has been validated for diagnosis of acute concussion, indicating the importance that this test be used as an adjunct to help guide clinical assessment.

King-Devick (K-D) Test

Question: Based on current literature, which diagnostic test is more appropriately applied in the clinic: King-Devick or VOMS?

The King-Devick (K-D) test is a rapid number naming test that is used as an objective way to assess saccadic eye movements and cognitive function. It can be performed using a computer/tablet-based application or printed flash cards. The athlete reads a series of numbers across horizontal rows that are spaced at different intervals across the page. The number sequences progressively increase in difficulty as the test goes on. The total time to complete the three test cards is recorded, and the number of errors is counted. This is compared to a baseline, which should be performed prior to concussion. Longer time to complete the test is a positive indicator for concussion.

The K-D test can be administered in about 2 min and has been studied most commonly as a sideline assessment to aid in the diagnosis of concussion. In recent years, the ability of this test to differentiate between concussed athletes and controls has been greatly debated. One study shows a sensitivity and specificity as high as 98% and 96%, respectively [6], while others show less favorable statistics with a sensitivity of 84% and a specificity of 62% [7]. It has also been shown to have diagnostic accuracy at 0–6 h and 24–48 h after injury [8], while other studies have shown less favorable outcomes. The K-D test does not seem to add unique information in diagnosing an acute concussion beyond what the SCAT can provide [9].

Due to the recent debate surrounding the accuracy of the K-D test in diagnosing acute concussion, it is advisable to use it in conjunction with other clinical exams. Some limitations include that it is a licensed product that does require a fee and a baseline test is recommended.

Sport Concussion Office Assessment Tool 6 (SCOAT6)

Question: What if the patient presents to your office several days after a concussion, is there a different evaluation that should be completed?

With the most recent 6th International Consensus Statement on Concussion in Sport [27], an additional office assessment tool was developed to aid healthcare professionals in the evaluation of sport-related concussion in an outpatient setting – the Sport Concussion Assessment Tool 6 (SCOAT6) [28]. It is designed to be used in a controlled office environment 72 hours to weeks after sport-related concussion for individuals aged 13 and older. There are several different sections, some of which are recommended in the evaluation and some of which are optional.

The recommended evaluation includes:

1. Patient demographics (focusing on history of head injuries and neuro/psychological diagnoses)
2. Symptom evaluation
3. Verbal cognitive tests (including immediate memory with ten-word recall, digits backwards, months in reverse order)
4. Orthostatic vital signs
5. Cervical spine and neurological assessment
6. Balance/coordination testing (including mBESS, timed tandem gait)
7. Modified vestibular/ocular motor screening (VOMS)
8. Delayed word recall

The optional sections include:

1. Complex tandem gait and dual task gait
2. Anxiety, depression, and sleep screening
3. Computerized cognitive test
4. Graded aerobic exercise test

While many of the individual components of the SCOAT6 have been validated on their own, the SCOAT6 as a multimodal assessment requires validation for use across various time points post-injury and in various patient populations/demographics [27].

This document is freely available for download and general use.

SCOAT6 (https://bjsm.bmj.com/content/bjsports/57/11/651.full.pdf)

Child SCOAT6

Question: Is there an alternative to SCOAT6 for younger children?

Similar to the SCAT6/child SCAT6 as above, there is an alternate version of the SCOAT6 for use in younger children [29]. The Child SCOAT6 is meant for use in children from 8 to 12 years of age in the outpatient clinic setting 72 hours to weeks after sport-related concussion. Compared with the SCOAT6, it includes a child-reported as well as parent-reported symptom evaluation, visio-vestibular examination instead of modified VOMS (mVOMS), and an optional symbol digit modalities test.

This document is freely available for download and general use.

Child SCOAT6 (https://bjsm.bmj.com/content/bjsports/57/11/672.full.pdf)

The Vestibular/Ocular Motor Screening (VOMS)

Question: Considering that the vestibular/ocular motor screening (VOMS) partly relies on the subjective report of the patient, how useful is it in the diagnosis of concussion?

Due to the multiple areas of the brain and vast number of neural connections that are involved with the vestibular and ocular systems, these areas are commonly affected in individuals who have sustained a concussion. In one study of pediatric patients, 81% showed an abnormality of the vestibular system on initial testing, and these athletes were shown to have longer time to return to school and play and also have lower scores on initial neurocognitive testing [10]. In another study, 69% of patients with a concussion had at least one visual abnormality, with 46% having impairment in more than one area [11].

The vestibular/ocular motor screening (VOMS) is a physical exam test to assess for impairments in the vestibular and ocular systems. It is a brief test that takes approximately 5–10 min to administer and generally consists of multiple components – smooth pursuits, horizontal and vertical saccades, horizontal and vertical vestibular ocular reflex (VOR), visual motion sensitivity (VMS), and near point convergence (NPC). The athlete is asked to report changes in four symptoms (headache, dizziness, nausea, and fogginess) compared to baseline using a number scale of 1–10 after each component. A visual depiction of this can be found at https://www.natafoundation.org/wp-content/uploads/VOMS-Infographic.pdf.

Impairment in any of the components of VOMS has been associated with concussion [30]. The test has high internal consistency and low false-positive rates as assessed in several recent studies [30–33]. In one study, an increase in ≥ 2 symptoms in any of the VOMS categories demonstrated a positive likelihood ratio of 23.9–42.8 in the diagnosis of concussion [30]. Utilizing the multiple components of VOMS increases its accuracy in detecting concussion, although recent studies have shown that NPC may not be as helpful as the other test categories [30, 34].

VOMS is a reliable, validated test for the evaluation of concussion. It is easy to perform in a short amount of time and does not depend on any additional tools. VOMS also does not require any baseline data, as a recent study demonstrated there was no increased diagnostic yield when compared with preseason testing [35]. Recent literature has demonstrated high reliability and low false-positive rates of VOMS. Thus, despite its dependency on subjective reporting of symptoms, it is a helpful test for use in the clinic to aid in the diagnosis of concussion. It has been validated for use in the clinic setting, but further research is needed to validate its use as a sideline tool. The VOMS is commonly included as part of the examination of a suspected concussion (also see the Physical Examination of Concussion Chapter for further details).

Orthostatic Vital Signs

Question: How does autonomic dysfunction manifest in orthostatic vital signs, and which measurement (BP or HR) is more important?

One of the early objective physiological signs of acute concussion is exercise intolerance, a manifestation believed to be related to impaired autonomic function. This belief is derived from studies that demonstrate a pattern of neurochemical and metabolic changes within the injured brain that result in physiologic changes largely controlled by the autonomic nervous system. The observed result, which has been confirmed across multiple studies, is an increase in sympathetic activity resulting in reduced heart rate variability, delayed blood pressure stabilization, and changes in cerebral perfusion [36, 37]. A simple, practical screening method for these physiologic changes in the clinic setting is measurement of orthostatic vital signs. Leddy et al. [14] describe using supine and standing (within 3 minutes) vital signs for the assessment of subjective and objective orthostatic intolerance. Subjectively, the patient may complain of dizziness, blurred vision, nausea, and/or feeling light-headed. The objective criteria is a 20 mm Hg drop of systolic blood pressure or a 10 mm Hg drop in diastolic blood pressure. In the setting of concussion evaluation, it is recommended to measure supine and standing only [38]. Heart rate is not required for the diagnosis but can be helpful in the clinical context; an increased heart rate (> 20 bpm) going from supine to standing may be reflective of hypovolemia, whereas a blunted HR response or lack of elevation is associated with neurogenic etiology [37, 38]. Athletes with a concussion may have orthostatic intolerance as demonstrated by symptoms alone and not meeting the objective criteria, thus demonstrating the importance of assessing symptom response to position changes and not just measuring the vital signs [39].

Notably, there is limited research that directly evaluates the diagnostic utility of orthostatic vital signs as it pertains to autonomic dysfunction for the evaluation of a concussion.

Buffalo Concussion Treadmill Test

Question: What is a standardized way to test physiologic dysfunction and exercise tolerance in concussed athletes?

The Buffalo Concussion Treadmill Test (BCTT) is a standardized protocol treadmill test that can be used in the diagnosis of acute concussion and recovery prognosis. A recent systematic review and meta-analysis found that exercise intolerance as evaluated using a graded exercise tolerance test (such as BCTT) has a 94% sensitivity and 95% specificity for the diagnosis of sport-related concussion [15]. It has evidence for use in developing a heart rate-based exercise plan for concussed athletes and/or assessing physiologic recovery. Recent research has shown that rest beyond the first couple of days after concussion can be detrimental rather than beneficial for recovery [40–42]. A recent randomized controlled trial of adolescent athletes showed that those who participated in progressive sub-symptom threshold aerobic exercise had a faster recovery than those assigned to a stretching program that did not raise their heart rate [43]. (See chapters on Concussion treatment and Concussion Return to Learn or Work and Return to Play for further details.)

The protocol (see Table 5.2) [40]:

The athlete is started at 3.6 mph at 0% incline. After the first minute, the incline is increased by 1% each minute. The athlete is assessed every minute for rating of perceived exertion (RPE, Borg scale) and for symptoms. Heart rate and blood pressure (if available) are monitored every 2 minutes. The test is stopped if the athlete has exacerbation of symptoms (≥ 3 points from pretest rating on 1- to 10-point visual analog scale) or at exhaustion (RPE of 19–20). If the maximal incline is reached without stopping criteria being met, the speed is increased by 0.4 mph every minute until stopping criteria are met. *The test should not be performed if the athlete has significant baseline symptoms of ≥ 7 on the pretest VAS.*

The BCTT has been shown to be a safe and reliable test of physiologic dysfunction in concussed athletes [40, 44]. With research continuing to support aerobic exercise in the recovery of concussed athletes, the BCTT provides an objective measurement of symptom threshold and can be used for patient-specific exercise recommendations [45]. The Buffalo Concussion Bike Test is an alternative that has been

Table 5.2 Buffalo concussion treadmill test [40]

Protocol	Starting speed is 3.6 mph at 0% incline Incline is increased by 1% each minute If maximum incline is reached and patient has not reached stoppage criteria, speed is increased by 0.4 mph each minute until stoppage criteria are met
Athlete monitoring	Rating of perceived exertion (RPE, Borg scale) and symptoms assessed each minute Heart rate and blood pressure measured every 2 min
Stoppage criteria	Significant exacerbation of symptoms (≥3 points from baseline that day on 1–10 point visual analog scale) OR At exhaustion (RPE of 19–20)

Contraindications to testing	Absolute:
	  Unwilling to exercise
	  Increased cardiac risk as defined by the American College of Sports Medicine
	  Focal neurologic deficit
	  Significant risk of walking/running on treadmill due to orthopedic injury, balance or visual deficit
	Relative:
	  Use of beta blockers
	  Major depression
	  Minor risk of walking/running on treadmill due to orthopedic injury, balance or visual deficit
	  SBP > 140 or DBP > 90
	  BMI ≥ 30

validated [46] and can be very useful if vestibular dysfunction, lower extremity injury, or limited mobility prohibit testing on the treadmill.

Biomarkers and Emerging Technologies

Question: Are there any laboratory tests that can be used to aid in the diagnosis of concussion?

As many of the diagnostic tests for concussion rely on subjective data, there is a need for more objective testing to help guide diagnosis. There are numerous ongoing research studies into the use of fluid-based biomarkers (saliva, blood, urine, cerebrospinal fluid), genetic tests, advanced neuroimaging, and other emerging technologies for diagnosis of concussion or predicting prognosis and recovery. A recent systematic review concluded that while many of these have shown sensitivity and utility in certain populations, the studies are small and lack generalizability [47]. Thus, the recommendation from the Concussion in Sport Group is that these remain helpful in the research of sport-related concussion but are not yet applicable in general practice [27]. With the increasing number of studies published over the recent years, these are areas that may soon be useful in the general population.

FDA-Approved Diagnostic Tests for Concussion

Question: My patient was asking about another diagnostic tool for concussion that they heard about on the news; are there any other FDA-approved tools to aid in the diagnosis of concussion?

Eye Tracking

Question: Are there any objective tests of ocular function that are not subject to human measurement?

It is well-known that patients with concussions have a high incidence of visual abnormalities, with one recent study reporting that 69% of adolescent athletes diagnosed with concussion had an abnormality in at least one visual test [11]. Developing reliable, objective tests for the diagnosis of concussion has been difficult. However, there has been recent evidence supporting the use of eye-tracking software to aid in the diagnosis of concussion. This can be a rapid, noninvasive way to test for concussion with the added benefit of not requiring a baseline test. A recent study reported a sensitivity of 57% and a specificity of 96% in the use of eye-tracking metrics for detection of convergence and accommodation abnormalities in a pediatric population with concussions [12]; other studies have confirmed a high sensitivity and specificity [48]. It has also been shown to have good test-retest reliability [49].

EyeBOX is a proprietary eye-tracking device that is FDA-approved for use in the diagnosis of concussion. It is a device that utilizes a unique algorithm to track eye movements while a patient watches a 4-min video clip. It is marketed for use in patients 5–67 years of age.

Eye-Sync is another device with FDA clearance as an aid to concussion that uses eye-tracking software to monitor eye movements to provide an objective way of measuring smooth pursuits, saccades, and VOR.

These devices provide more objective data in the diagnosis of concussion that helps to minimize the human measurement factor. However, they require the use of proprietary software and thus can be expensive and are not readily available in the general primary care clinic.

The most recent sports concussion consensus guidelines note the research in this area under the umbrella of "emerging technologies." There are several devices and technologies in this field, and, as always, more research is needed.

Force Plate/BTrackS/Sway Balance

Question: Is there a more objective test of balance than the BESS test?

Balance testing is an evidence-based recommended component in the complete concussion evaluation [50]. BESS is the standard of balance testing, but due to its relatively low sensitivity and subjective nature, there is a need for a more sensitive and objective test. Standard force plate technology has been the gold standard of balance testing but can be expensive and requires high-tech equipment. BTrackS is a relatively low-cost alternative force plate that provides a higher sensitivity than BESS at 64% while still having high specificity at 90% [13]. It has also been shown to have high test-retest reliability, and there is no practice improvement with repeat testing [51]. It is a rapid (<2 min), portable, objective measure of balance.

SWAY is a FDAP-cleared class II application available for Apple and Android tablets or phones that uses accelerometer data to objectively measure an athlete's balance while performing BESS testing. Studies have validated the accuracy and reliability of its data with high-tech force plates [52], but there is recent research questioning the convergent validity of SWAY in concussed cadets [53]. SWAY is an objective tool for measuring balance and it can be done virtually via smartphone.

There are several other force plate products each with different profiles in terms of precision, accuracy, feasibility, and cost. This is outside the scope of this chapter.

Key Points

- The Post-Concussion Symptom Scale has the highest diagnostic utility when used within 3–5 days post-injury and may help prognosticate duration of recovery.
- The SCAT6 (and Child SCAT6) integrate several components (PCSS, SAC, mBESS) into one evaluation that is most reliable when used within 3 days post-injury.
- The SCAT6 (and Child SCAT6) are tools that can be used in the office to aid in the diagnosis of concussion. They cannot be completed in less than 10–15 minutes and should be used within 3 days (ideally) but up to 7 days post-concussion.
- The SCOAT6 and Child SCOAT6 are similar to the SCAT6 but are designed to be used in the outpatient setting from 3 to 30 days after concussion.
- Both the BESS and mBESS evaluate for static postural instability and rely on the subjective assessment of the observer.
- Orthostatic vital signs can be a useful diagnostic test to identify orthostatic intolerance and/or autonomic dysfunction after a concussion.
- VOMS is a reliable, validated test for the evaluation of concussion. No baseline is required, and there is no cost to perform the test, making this feasible and practical for most clinicians.
- The Buffalo Concussion Treadmill Test is a safe and reliable way to test for physiologic dysfunction in the concussed athlete; it is commonly used to help determine symptom threshold and guide return to activity recommendations.
- Biomarkers, neuroimaging, and advanced technologies are helpful as research tools but are not yet generalizable for use in clinical practice

References

1. Resch JE, Brown CN, Schmidt J, et al. The sensitivity and specificity of clinical measures of sport concussion: three tests are better than one. BMJ Open SEM. 2016;2:e000012. https://doi.org/10.1136/bmjsem-2015-000012.
2. Echemendia RJ, Burma JS, Bruce JM, Davis GA, Giza CC, Guskiewicz KM, Naidu D, Black AM, Broglio S, Kemp S, Patricios JS, Putukian M, Zemek R, Arango-Lasprilla JC, Bailey CM, Brett BL, Didehbani N, Gioia G, Herring SA, Howell D, Master CL, Valovich McLeod TC, Meehan WP 3rd, Premji Z, Salmon D, van Ierssel J, Bhathela N, Makdissi M, Walton SR, Kissick J, Pardini J, Schneider KJ. Acute evaluation of sport-related concussion and implications for the Sport Concussion Assessment Tool (SCAT6) for adults, adolescents and children: a systematic review. Br J Sports Med. 2023;57(11):722–35. https://doi.org/10.1136/bjsports-2022-106661.
3. Standardized Assessment of Concussion. Newburgh City School District. Retrieved from https://www.newburghschools.org/files/departments/athletics/ConcussionTestForm.pdf. last accessed 31 October 2019.
4. Sport Concussion Assessment Tool 6. British Journal of Sports Medicine. Retrieved from https://bjsm.bmj.com/content/bjsports/57/11/622.full.pdf

5. Military Acute Concussion Evaluation 2. The Defense and Veterans Brain Injury Center. Retrieved from: https://www.health.mil/Reference-Center/Publications/2020/07/30/Military-Acute-Concussion-Evaluation-MACE-2

6. Hecimovich M, King D, Dempsey AR, et al. The King-Devick test is a valid and reliable tool for assessing sport-related concussion in Australian football: a prospective cohort study. J Sci Med Sport. 2018;21:1004–7. https://doi.org/10.1016/j.jsams.2018.03.011.

7. Naidu D, Borza C, Kobitowich T, et al. Sideline concussion assessment: the King-Devick test in Canadian professional football. J Neurotrauma. 2018;35:2283–6. https://doi.org/10.1089/neu.2017.5490.

8. Le RK, Ortega J, Chrisman SP, Kontos AP, Buckley TA, Kaminski TW, Meyer BP, Clugston JR, Goldman JT, McAllister T, McCrea M, Broglio SP, Schmidt JD. King-Devick sensitivity and specificity to concussion in collegiate athletes. J Athl Train. 2023;58(2):97–105. https://doi.org/10.4085/1062-6050-0063.21.

9. Echemendia RJ, Thelen J, Meeuwisse W, et al. The utility of the King-Devick test in evaluating professional ice hockey players with suspected concussion. Clin J Sport Med. 2022;32:265–71. https://doi.org/10.1097/JSM.0000000000000841.

10. Corwin DJ, Wiebe DJ, Zonfrillo MR, Grady MF, Robinson RL, Goodman AM, Master CL. Vestibular deficits following youth concussion. J Pediatr. 2015;166(5):1221–5.

11. Master CL, Schieman M, Gallaway M, Goodman A, Robinson RL, Master SR, Grady MF. Vision diagnoses are common after concussion in adolescents. Clin Pediatr. 2016;55(3):260–7.

12. Bin Zahid A, Hubbard ME, Lockyer J, Podolak O, Dammavalam VM, Grady M, Nance M, Schieman M, Samadani U, Master CL. Eye tracking as a biomarker for concussion in children. Clin J Sport Med. 2018;

13. Goble DJ, Manyak KA, Abdenour TE, Rauh MJ, Baweja HS. An initial evaluation of the BTrackS balance plate and sports balance software for concussion diagnosis. Int J Sports Phys Ther. 2016;11(2):149–55.

14. Leddy J, Baker JG, Haider MN, Hinds A, Willer B. A physiological approach to prolonged recovery from sport-related concussion. J Athl Train. 2017;52(3):299–308. https://doi.org/10.4085/1062-6050-51.11.08.

15. Haider MN, Lutnick E, Nazir MSZ, Nowak A, Chizuk HM, Miecznikowski JC, McPherson JI, Willer BS, Leddy JJ. Sensitivity and specificity of exercise intolerance on graded exertion testing for diagnosing sport-related concussion: a systematic review and exploratory meta-analysis. J Neurotrauma. 2023;40(15-16):1524–32. https://doi.org/10.1089/neu.2022.0331. Epub 2023 Jun 5

16. Meehan WP 3rd, O'Brien MJ, Geminiani E, Mannix R. Initial symptom burden predicts duration of symptoms after concussion. J Sci Med Sport. 2015;19(9):722–5.

17. Harmon KG, Clugston JR, Dec K, et al. American medical society for sports medicine position statement on concussion in sport. Br J Sports Med. 2019;53:213–25.

18. Karr JE, Zuccato BG, Ingram EO, McAuley TL, Merker B, Abeare CA. The post-concussion symptom scale: normative data for adolescent student-athletes stratified by gender and preexisting conditions. Am J Sports Med. 2023;51(1):225–36. https://doi.org/10.1177/03635465221131987. Epub 2022 Nov 25

19. Dessy AM, Yuk FJ, Maniya AY, Gometz A, Rasouli J, et al. Review of assessment scales for diagnosing and monitoring sports-related concussion. Cureus. 2017;9(12):–e1922.

20. Hecht S, Puffer J, Clinton C, Aish B, Cohen P, Concoff A, et al. Concussion assessment in football and soccer players. Clin J Sport Med. 2004;14:310.

21. Van Deventer KA, Seehusen CN, Walker GA, et al. The diagnostic and prognostic utility of the dual-task Tandem gait test for pediatric concussion. J Sport Health Sci. 2021;10:131–7. https://doi.org/10.1016/j.jshs.2020.08.005.

22. Child Sport Concussion Assessment Tool 6. British Journal of Sports Medicine. Retrieved from https://bjsm.bmj.com/content/bjsports/57/11/636.full.pdf

23. Davis GA, Echemendia RJ, Ahmed OH, et al. Introducing the child sport concussion assessment tool 6 (Child SCAT6). Br J Sports Med. 2023;57:632–5.

24. Davis GA, Purcell L, Schneider KJ, Yeates KO, Gioia GA, et al. the child sport concussion assessment tool 5th Edition (Child SCAT5): background and rationale. Br J Sports Med. 2017;51(11):859–61.
25. Stone ME, Safadjou S, Farber B, Velazco N, Man J, et al. Utility of the military acute concussion evaluation as a screening tool for mild traumatic brain injury in a civilian trauma population. J Trauma Acute Care Surgery. 2015;79(1):147–51.
26. Khokhar B, Jorgensen-Wagers K, Marion D, Kiser S. Military acute concussion evaluation: a report on clinical usability, utility and user's perceived confidence. J Neurotrauma. 2021;38(2):210–2017. https://doi.org/10.1089/neu.2020.7176.
27. Consensus Statement on Concussion in Sport: the 6th International Conference on Concussion in Sport–Amsterdam, 2022. British Journal of Sports Medicine https://bjsm.bmj.com/content/bjsports/57/11/695.full.pdf
28. Sport Concussion Office Assessment Tool 6. British Journal of Sports Medicine. Retrieved from https://bjsm.bmj.com/content/bjsports/57/11/651.full.pdf
29. Child Sport Concussion Office Assessment Tool 6. British Journal of Sports Medicine. Retrieved from https://bjsm.bmj.com/content/bjsports/57/11/672.full.pdf
30. Mucha A, Collins MW, Elbin RJ, Furman JM, Troutman-Enseki C, DeWolf RM, Marchetti G, Kontos AP. A brief vestibular/ocular motor screening (VOMS) assessment to evaluate concussions. Am J Sports Med. 2014;42(10):2479–86.
31. Worts PR, Schatz P, Burkhart SO. Test performance and test-retest reliability of the vestibular/ocular motor screening and King-Devick test in adolescent athletes during a competitive sport season. Am J Sports Med. 2018;46(8):2004–10.
32. Moran RN, Covassin T, Elbin RJ, Gould D, Nogle S. Reliability and normative reference values for the vestibular/ocular motor screening (VOMS) tool in youth athletes. Am J Sports Med. 2018;46(6):1475–80.
33. Rosenblum D, Donahue C, Higgins H, Brna M, Resch J. False-positive rates, risk factors, and interpretations of the vestibular ocular motor screen in collegiate athletes. J Athl Train. 2023; https://doi.org/10.4085/1062-6050-0317.23.
34. Apps J, Walter K, editors. Pediatric and adolescent concussion: diagnosis, management, and outcomes. New York: Springer; 2012.
35. Ferris LM, Kontos AP, Eagle SR, Elbin RJ, Collins MW, Mucha A, McAllister TW, Broglio SP, McCrea M, Pasquina PF, Port NL. Utility of VOMS, SCAT3, and ImPACT Baseline evaluations for acute concussion identification in collegiate athletes: findings from the NCAA-DoD concussion assessment, research and education (CARE) consortium. Am J Sports Med. 2022;50(4):1106–19. https://doi.org/10.1177/03635465211072261. Epub 2022 Feb 18
36. Leddy J, Kozlowski K, Fung M, Pendergast DR, Willer B. Regulatory and autoregulatory physiological dysfunction as a primary characteristic of post concussion syndrome: implications for treatment. Neuro Rehabilitation. 2007;22(3):199–205.
37. Pertab JL, Merkley TL, Cramond AJ, Cramond K, Paxton H, et al. Concussion and the autonomic nervous system: an introduction to the field and the results of a systematic review. Neuro Rehabilitation. 2018;42(4):397–427.
38. Matuszak JM, McVige J, McPherson J, Willer B, Leddy J. A practical concussion physical examination toolbox. Sports Health. 2016;8(3):260–9. https://doi.org/10.1177/1941738116641394.
39. Haider MN, Patel KS, Willer BS, Videira V, Wilber CG, Mayer AR, Master CL, Mariotti BL, Wertz C, Storey EP, Arbogast KB, Park G, Oglesbee SJ, Bezherano I, Aguirre K, Fodero JG, Johnson BD, Mannix R, Miecznikowski JC, Leddy JJ. Symptoms upon postural change and orthostatic hypotension in adolescents with concussion. Brain Inj. 2021;35(2):226–32. https://doi.org/10.1080/02699052.2021.1871951.
40. Leddy JJ, Willer B. Use of graded exercise testing in concussion and return-to-activity management. Cur Sports Med Reports. 2013;12(6):370–6.
41. Leddy JJ, Wilber CG, Willer B. Active recovery from concussion. Curr Opin Neurol. 2018;31(6):681–6.

42. Lawrence DW, Richards D, Comper P, Hutchinson MG. Earlier time to aerobic exercise is asso-ciated with faster recovery following acute sport concussion. PLoS One. 2018;13(4):e0196062.
43. Leddy JJ, Haider MN, Ellis MJ, Mannix R, Darling SR, Freitas MS, Suffoletto HN, Leiter J, Cordingley DM, Willer B. Early subthreshold aerobic exercise for sport-related concussion: a randomized clinical trial. JAMA Pediatr. 2019;173(4):319–25.
44. Leddy JJ, Hinds AL, Miecznikowski J, Darling S, Matuszak J, Baker JG, Picano J, Willer B. Safety and prognostic utility of provocative exercise testing in acutely concussed adoles-cents: a randomized trial. Clin J Sport Med. 2018;28(1):13–20.
45. Leddy J, Hinds A, Sirica D, Willer B. The role of controlled exercise in concussion manage-ment. PM&R. 2016;8(35):S91–S100.
46. Haider MN, Johnson SL, Mannix R, Macfarlane AJ, Constantino D, Johnson BD, Leddy J. The Buffalo concussion bike test for concussion assessment in adolescents. Sports Health. 2019; https://doi.org/10.1177/1941738119870189.
47. Tabor JB, Brett BL, Nelson L, Meier T, Penner LC, Mayer AR, Echemendia RJ, McAllister T, Meehan WP, Patricios J, Makdissi M. Role of biomarkers and emerging technologies in defin-ing and assessing neurobiological recovery after sport-related concussion: a systematic review. Br J Sports Med. 2023;57(12):789–97.
48. Samadani U, Li M, Qian M, Laska E, Ritlop R, Kolecki R, Reyes M, Altomare L, Yeong Sone J, Adem A, Huang P, Kondziolka D, Wall S, Frangos S, Marmar C. Sensitivity and specificity of an eye movement tracking-based biomarker for concussion. Concussion. 2016;1(1):CNC3.
49. Howell DR, Brilliant AN, Master CL, Meehan WP. Reliability of objective eye-tracking mea-sures among healthy adolescent athletes. Clin J Sport Med. 2018;
50. Harmon KG, Clugston JR, Dec K, Hainline B, Herring SA, Kane S, Kontos AP, Leddy JJ, McCrea MA, Poddar SK, Putukian M, Wilson JC, Roberts WO. American medical soci-ety for sports medicine position statement on concussion in sport. Clin J Sport Med. 2019;29(2):87–100.
51. Hearn M, Levy S, Baweja H, Goble D. BTrackS balance test for concussion management is resistant to practice effects. Clin J Sport Med. 2018;28(2):177–9.
52. Dabbs NC, Sauls NM, Zayer A, Chander H. Balance performance in collegiate athletes: a comparison of balance error scoring system measures. J Funct Morphol Kinesiol. 2017;2(26)
53. Dummar MK, Crowell MS, Pitt W, Yu AM, McHenry P, Benedict T, Morris J, Miller EM. The convergent validity of the SWAY balance application to assess postural stability in military cadets recovering from concussion. Int J Sports Phys Ther. 2024;19(2):166–75.

Chapter 6
Concussion Neurocognitive Testing

Jeffrey M. Mjaanes and J. Matthew Nerrie

Clinical Case

A 14-year-old high school basketball player is seeking clearance from a concussion sustained 12 days ago. Her somatic symptoms resolved within a few days, but she reports some slight difficulties with memory recall on homework. She took a baseline cognitive test before the season but does not have the results of the test, and you do not have access to the system. You are considering how best to evaluate her neurocognitive status.

What is the difference between neuropsychological and neurocognitive testing?

The term "neurocognitive" testing is often used interchangeably with "neuropsychological" testing, but there are subtle differences. Neurocognitive testing can fall under the larger umbrella term of neuropsychological testing but refers to specific measures of cognition. These measures typically include short- and long-term memory, attention, language, visuospatial skills, cognitive processing speed, and executive functions like response inhibition [1]. Neuropsychological testing examines the psychological functioning of personality, mood, depression, as well as sensory and motor functions.

While both approaches to testing are used to evaluate the relationship between the brain and behavior, there are significant differences in the scope of use, information derived, cost, evaluation time, and usefulness in neurorehabilitation planning. A neuropsychological examination performed by a trained neuropsychologist is the gold standard for assessing all areas of brain function and includes a comprehensive evaluation of sensory/motor function, auditory and visual attention, working memory, verbal and visual memory, language, executive function, speed of processing,

J. M. Mjaanes (✉) · J. M. Nerrie
Northwestern Medicine, Evanston, IL, USA
e-mail: jmjaanes@northwestern.edu; Jeffrey.mjaanes@nm.org; Matt.nerrie@nm.org

intellectual ability, and emotional capacity. The examination is multidimensional and employs a combination, or battery, of tests that can produce a composite score across multiple ability areas and provide an overall index of how well a person functions cognitively at the time of testing [2]. As a result, testing is time-consuming, lasting several hours which may even be spread out over several days depending on the referral question and information needed. The results are referenced to demographic groups of age, sex, race, and education levels. There are also internal checks to determine an examinee's effort and testing validity. The results are typically interpreted by psychologists, neuropsychologists, or neuropsychiatrists and compared against known deficit profiles related to illness, disease, and injury for diagnosis. The results are detailed enough to be used for neurorehabilitation planning, special education placement, competency determination, forensic/legal purposes, drug or treatment research, mental/behavioral health screening, and identification of functional impairments. Many of the various testing instruments were developed before the widespread use of computers and are administered using paper, pencil, and a stopwatch. In recent years there have been concerted efforts to computerize many of these tests, which require lengthy re-standardization processes. Traditional pencil-and-paper tests include those seen in Table 6.1. Most of these tests are copyright-protected and require advance training and licensing to purchase, administer, and interpret. Most experts recommend the test be administered or at least supervised by a licensed psychologist, usually a board-certified neuropsychologist with clinical experience in evaluating sports-related concussion [2, 3].

Alternatively, neurocognitive testing is aimed at addressing a subset of symptoms or cognitive functions related to a particular illness or injury. Many of these tests were created purposefully for computer use to facilitate ease of administration, portability, and rapid scoring; some even include basic interpretation and provide limited age-related norms. The SAC, ImPACT, Concussion Vital Signs, ANAM, Axon, C3 Logix, and other neurocognitive testing platforms were designed and standardized to quickly assess cognitive deficits seen with concussion, emphasizing

Table 6.1 Common neuropsychological tests used in sports concussion assessments[a]

Neuropsychological test	Cognitive domain
Controlled oral word association (COWAT)	Verbal fluency
Hopkins verbal learning test	Verbal learning, immediate and delayed memory
Paced auditory serial addition test	Attention, concentration
Stroop color word test	Attention, information processing speed
Symbol digit modalities test	Psychomotor speed, attention, concentration
Trail making: parts A & B	Visual scanning, attention, information processing speed, psychomotor speed
Weschler adult intelligence scale	Intelligence and cognitive ability
Wechsler digit span: digits forward and backward	Concentration, attention
Wechsler letter numbering sequencing test	Verbal working memory

[a]Typically administered in a one-on-one testing environment

attention, processing speed, and memory. However, these devices could be inappropriate and even invalid in the evaluation of other cognitive impairments including learning disability, ADHD, brain tumor, stroke, traumatic brain injury, and other neurological conditions, due to limited domain assessment, differing comparison groups, and interpretation by those not qualified to provide a medical or psychological diagnosis. A benefit is the administration of neurocognitive testing can be done by nonphysician medical staff. Some offer tablet-based administration for complete portability and provide cloud storage for universal wireless access. The healthcare provider will want to become familiar with administration and interpretation documentation, especially if there are questions or concerns about effort that may impact activity progression or returning to play. The commercially available CNT have disclaimers that they should not be used as the sole determinant for diagnosing or return to play decision for concussions. Lingering recovery due to comorbidities or worrisome cognitive deficits may require a more comprehensive assessment and can always be referred for a full neuropsychological examination.

Question: What single test can reliably confirm the diagnosis of concussion?

The clinical diagnosis of concussion can be challenging. At times a concussion may be readily apparent, for example, a loss of consciousness or seizure after obvious forceful head impact. However, frequently the presentation can be ambiguous and the diagnosis unclear. For example, the inciting trauma or mechanism of injury may appear benign, the symptoms may be mild or delayed in onset, and other objective signs may be lacking. Some injured athletes may present with deficits in balance and vision, while other athletes may have no balance or visual challenges but instead have cognitive and sleep disturbances. Given the variety of clinical manifestations, the 2022 Concussion in Sport Group recommends a multimodal evaluation for concussion in athletes, including assessment of the following domains: symptoms, signs, balance, gait, neurological function, and cognition [4].

Standard structural neuroimaging, such as computerized tomography or magnetic resonance imaging, is normal in concussion as there is no gross anatomical disturbance. Functional blood flow or neurometabolic imaging studies, like functional magnetic resonance imaging, are useful in research settings investigating concussion, but their clinical use is so far limited as additional studies are needed to demonstrate clinical validity [5]. Multiple studies have identified blood biomarkers that rise and fall during a concussion marking the metabolic changes following this injury; [6] however, no individual biomarker or combination of these biomarkers has yet been proven a reliable and definitive test to rule in or rule out a concussion. Further details may be found in the Concussion Imaging and Concussion Diagnostic Testing chapters.

As noted in previous chapters, concussion can present with a wide variety of symptoms and clinical findings spread over several different physical, emotional, and cognitive domains. Therefore, a thorough evaluation for concussion should contain elements that provide information from each of these domains. Neuropsychological testing can provide important and useful information on the cognitive and emotional domains.

Question: Is neuropsychological testing a new development?

Attempts at trying to localize cognitive functions in the brain started early in the history of medicine. Herophilus is often given credit for first attempting this evaluation process in 300 B.C [7]. After World War II, advances in neuropsychology were achieved through the work of Alexander Luria, Anne-Lise Christensen, Arthur Benton, and others [8]. Originally the primary objective of neuropsychological testing was to identify brain dysfunction, but in more recent years, the role of repeat evaluations has emerged with the goal of monitoring disease progression or recovery.

Computerized neurocognitive testing (CNT) is a relatively recent development allowing for a more concise assessment of certain domains of cognitive function. The first computerized neurocognitive test batteries became commercially available in the mid-1990s [8]. The advent of portable computer devices such as smartphones and tablets has continued to enhance the ability to access neurocognitive assessments in diverse settings, including on sport sidelines. These advances have reduced the equipment requirements and improved access to testing.

Question: Are computer-based neurocognitive tests a viable option in concussion evaluation?

Computerized neurocognitive testing (CNT) has been considered an integral component of concussion assessments for the last 10–15 years [4, 9, 10]. As mentioned above, traditional neuropsychological testing provides a more comprehensive assessment of neurological, cognitive, and emotional conditions; however, time and resource constraints in sports medicine often favor more concise and focused neurocognitive assessments of cognitive domains most often affected by concussion (e.g., memory, attention, processing speed, and reaction time). Computerized assessments can now be performed on tablets or smart phones, increasing their portability, accessibility, and ease of use. While computerized testing may not yield as much information as full neuropsychological evaluation, they can provide more objective information to aid clinical decision-making for a suspected concussion.

The consensus statements published by the Concussion in Sport Group (CISG) have evolved in their recommendations around use and interpretation of neurocognitive testing in sports-related concussion (SRC). The most recent CISG consensus statement from the 2022 International Conference on Concussion in Sport in Amsterdam states that neurocognitive tests, where accessible, may add value to assessing SRC and its sequelae, especially when comparing post-injury reaction times against patient baseline and community normative values. The CISG made particular note that the results of these tests should be interpreted in the context of broader clinical findings and computerized test results should not be used to inform management or diagnostic decisions in isolation but should be part of a broader multimodal evaluation.

Question: What are some of the benefits of computerized neurocognitive testing?

Computerized neurocognitive assessments have found an increasingly common role in the evaluation and assessment of sports-related concussion. Different forms of these tests have increased in use for many reasons including practicality, ease of interpretation, and portability. The companies producing the CNTs suggest and inform on how to administer and interpret the tests, but no formal training or certification is required. Tests can be administered by downloading an application or accessing the platform via web-based portals. Newer tablet-based tests have improved the portability, making it possible to take the test in nearly any environment. The results can then be uploaded to a central server allowing for review from any computer with web access. For example, these tests can be administered by a certified athletic trainer (AT) on a sideline and then be remotely reviewed by a physician.

Computer-based neurocognitive assessment tools (Table 6.2) are much less time-consuming, often taking 10–30 min to complete, when compared to a traditional 4-h neuropsychological test battery. These tests also differ from traditional neuropsychological testing in that they do not need to be administered or interpreted by a certified testing specialist. Scoring for these computer-based tests is automated and often produces a summary sheet for statistical analysis or automatically compared to baseline and/or age-related normative data.

These computer-based neurocognitive tests are useful for large group baseline testing, often performed at the time of sport pre-participation examinations or pre-season. With the relative ease of baseline testing, post-injury evaluations can readily be compared to the baseline test for an individual athlete and performed serially to assess for progression/recovery [11]. A baseline comparison is particularly useful in those cases where learning or testing difficulties (ADHD, dyslexia, etc.) and other confounding diagnoses, such as depression or chronic migraine, can interfere with normative test data. Another unique benefit to these computerized test batteries is that they allow for accurate and quantified measurements of reaction time, [3, 12, 13] which is more difficult to obtain at the same level of accuracy on paper-and-pencil assessments. One of the final benefits of computer-based tests is the number of controlled test variations for serial testing. It may be more difficult to maintain the number of variations to accomplish this same task in traditional paper and pencil tests [11]. Multiple retest variations are important for the athlete that is retaking tests over a relatively short time frame in order to track recovery and aid return to play decisions in an active management program.

Question: What is the role for computerized neurocognitive testing on the field side for possible concussions and how does the field-side assessment differ from the evaluation in the clinic?

CNTs have increased in use and form part of many formal professional, collegiate, and high school concussion protocols because they can be administered relatively quickly and be performed as part of a baseline and post-injury assessment.

Table 6.2 Computerized neurocognitive assessments

Test	Measured subtests	Summary scores
ANAM (Automated Neuropsychological Assessment Metrics)	Simple reaction time Procedural reaction time Code substitution learning Code substitution delayed Mathematical processing Matching to sample Second administration	Standardized subtest Standardized composite Composite score Classification of Impairment
AXON CogState	Processing speed Attention Learning Working memory	Subtest summary scores Composite score Classification of impairment
C3Logix	Symbol digit coding Simple reaction time Choice reaction time Trails A & B Verbal memory test, immediate Verbal memory test, delayed SAC Concentration	Processing speed Inter-symbol response time and accuracy Simple reaction time Choice reaction time Trails A time Trails B time Trails B minus A time Immediate memory Delayed memory SAC composite score
CNS Vital Signs	Verbal memory test, immediate Visual memory test, immediate Finger tapping test Symbol digit coding Stroop test Shifting attention test Continuous performance test Verbal memory test, delayed Visual memory test, delayed	Neurocognitive index Composite memory Verbal memory Visual memory Psychomotor speed Reaction time Complex attention Cognitive flexibility Processing speed Executive function Simple attention Motor speed Composite score: IQ
HeadMinder (CRI)	Reaction Time Cued reaction time Visual recognition 1 & 2 Animal decoding Symbol Scanning	Psychomotor Speed index Simple reaction time
ImPACT	Word memory, immediate Design memory, immediate X's and O's Symbol match Color match Four letters Word memory, delayed Design memory, delayed	Verbal memory Visual memory Visual motor speed Reaction Time Impulse control

Table 6.3 Modified
Maddocks questions
from SCAT 6

| What venue are we at today? |
| What half is it now? |
| Who scored last in this match? |
| What team did you play last week/game? |
| Did your team win the last game? |

However, the requirement of a field-side test is different from a more detailed clinical assessment. Even a 10- to 30-min CNT does not have a role in the immediate field-side evaluation. Field-side assessment is used to evaluate an athlete and establish some validation of a concussion injury. A concussion injury is defined as a traumatic brain injury caused by a direct blow to the head, neck, or body resulting in an impulsive force being transmitted to the brain [4]. The decision to return an athlete to the field of play can be difficult, and there can be pressure to make it rapidly. In many cases, the signs and symptoms of a concussion evolve over a number of minutes to hours and occasionally days [9]. Therefore, if the athlete shows enough evidence for a possible diagnosis of concussion during the assessment, they must be removed from play for the rest of that day. A more complete assessment can then be performed at a later time. Neurocognitive testing and even typical CNTs have limited clinical utility in making the immediate, sideline decisions for a concussion injury. The need for immediate decision-making on the sideline has been the motivation for the development of several brief assessment tools. The functionality of these tests differs from both the traditional neuropsychological test batteries and the more recent CNTs. Brief field-side neurocognitive tests include the paper and pencil Standardized Assessment of Concussion (SAC) and the Sports Concussion Assessment Tool 6 (SCAT6) which includes modified Maddocks questions [4] (see Table 6.3). More recently, some applications such as C3Logix and ImPACT Quick Test have incorporated similar components of these paper-and-pencil brief field-side assessments into a digital format on a computer tablet.

Question: What are some concerns about using computerized neurocognitive testing?

While CNTs may have numerous advantages, several criticisms have also been raised, especially from within the neuropsychology community. One preeminent concern is the limited test-retest reliability and variable sensitivity of computer-based neurocognitive testing. A recent head-to-head comparison of three commercially available CNTs, found the test-retest reliability was similar among the three platforms but that it was below optimal standards for clinical use on many subtests [14]. Reliability refers to the consistency of the scores obtained from a test and whether the results can be reproduced under similar conditions. In concussion testing, reliability is relevant given the individual, serial nature of testing over time, from baseline when applicable, through post-injury assessments. Interpretation relies on evaluation of differences in post-injury performance compared to either baseline, prior post-injury test, or age-stratified norms, with the assumption that the differences in scores are due to the injury. If a test has a low-reliability coefficient, it may be difficult to attribute the testing result changes to the injury. Reliability has been highly variable in CNT studies, with reliability coefficients shown to be uniformly poor in some samples and stronger in others [14].

To reduce measurement errors, many CNT systems calculate a reliable change index, or RCI, which estimates the magnitude of differences in scores necessary to suggest true change. When reliability is low, the RCI will be high and vice versa. When comparing three CNT systems, Nelson and colleagues found that the sensitivity of RCIs was best at 24 h but diminished to near the false-positive rates in non-injured controls afterward [14]. Sensitivities were highest in athletes who became asymptomatic within 1 day before testing, but for those who became asymptomatic earlier, sensitivity was closer to the test's false-positive rate. The authors concluded that CNTs may add incrementally beyond symptom scores to the identification of clinical impairment within 24 h of injury or within a brief period after symptom resolution but do not add significant value over symptoms assessment later. In other words, CNTs tend to demonstrate the ability to distinguish between concussed and non-concussed athletes during the early stages post-injury, but their clinical utility later appears limited [15].

Other concerns regarding CNTs have emphasized lack of standardization of what is being studied and that much of the research has been industry-sponsored. Each commercially available CNT uses different testing formats to assess the cognitive domains they deem most important. Not all tested domains are the same, and even for those whose measured domains are similar, differences in the specific subsets are enough to make direct comparisons difficult if not impossible [14]. Additionally, there is no consensus among concussion experts on the protocols for use of CNTs, or which measures, or combination of measures, best differentiate concussed from non-concussed athletes. Lastly, much of the research in the field of CNTs has been conducted by the industry itself, including the companies that developed the tests. There is a paucity of peer reviewed research directly comparing the performance of the currently available CNTs.

Question: What do you do if the patient didn't complete a baseline test or lack access to baseline testing results?

In any clinic environment, there will be many concussion cases that present without baseline testing data. In these cases, normative data comparison is used for scoring the testing results. Commercially available CNTs have their own normative database; however, some care should be taken using normative data comparisons. Traditional neuropsychological tests have normative data sets typically grouped by age in 5-year blocks from ages 18–89. Newer CNTs do not necessarily use the groupings; therefore you must have a deep understanding of the tool you are using to ensure as close to an apples-to-apples comparison as possible. Performance on baseline and post-injury testing can be affected by many factors including sleep habits, medication usage and timing, underlying mental health concerns, and fueling patterns. There can be a significant difference in performance norms especially in the younger and older populations as cognitive abilities develop or decline, respectively. Baseline testing is already part of many organizational concussion protocols as it can assist a managing clinician in assessing injury status and recovery from injury but is no longer considered an integral part of concussion management [16].

Question: Can an athlete purposefully give poor effort during baseline testing or "sandbag" in order to return to play more quickly after a concussion?

Even with an optimal pretest screening and testing environment, the test taker's effort can significantly affect testing results. It has been suggested that athletes may provide suboptimal effort, sometimes called "sandbagging," in order to return to their baseline cognitive scores and return to play more quickly [17]. Traditional lengthy neuropsychological test batteries contain built-in measures to assess performance validity. These measures can be useful in understanding performance inconsistencies from comorbid conditions but are also useful in picking up effort-related inconsistencies. The more commonly used CNTs do not employ all the same measures as classical neuropsychological testing to evaluate performance, but several tests use internal validity indicators in a similar fashion. These measures are designed to identify results that may have been adversely affected by many factors including suboptimal effort, but much of the research on these measures has been industry-sponsored. One study showed 11% of ImPACT savvy college athletes were able to successfully "sandbag" a baseline ImPACT test without activating the test internal validity indicators [18]. Another study showed 30% of ImPACT-naïve nonathlete college students were able to "sandbag" without being caught by the ImPACT validity indicators [19].

Traditional neuropsychological tests are administered and interpreted one-on-one. Even though CNTs may be administered to many people at one time, baseline testing must be reviewed and examined one test at a time for valid results. In a survey of athletic trainers in 2009 reviewing the use of ImPACT testing, only 55% examined baselines for valid results [20]. If the baseline test is invalid, it cannot reliably be used for comparison as part of the return to play decision-making process.

Question: Why do I have to use a wired mouse with some tests when I normally use a wireless mouse with my computer?

Rapid evolution of computer systems continues to play a role in the usability and portability of neurocognitive tests. Computer-based testing has evolved as technology has advanced. Testing just a few years ago on desktop systems with wired components evolved to testing on portable laptop systems with Bluetooth or wireless components. Some neurocognitive assessments now utilize portable tablets and cell phones for testing. One of the advantages of the computer-based neurocognitive testing batteries has been the ability of a computer to assess subtests, such as reaction time, to an exceedingly small and sensitive level. Establishing a valid normative database for subtests such as reaction time requires specific and standardized computer hardware configurations. The power of large normative databases arises from the number of the same tests with the same hardware configurations stored and available for reference. Changing even one component, such as a wired mouse for a Bluetooth wireless mouse, can affect the sensitive results and ultimately challenge the integrity of the normative database. It is difficult for neurocognitive testing systems to keep up with the rapid advances in technology. Newer tests are coming to market on current technology, but even these may be outdated as technology advances. Traditionally, ImPACT testing system requires a desktop or laptop computer with a wired mouse (not wireless or Bluetooth mouse) to assure correlation with their normative database but has since developed normative databases for trackpads. External wireless devices are discouraged as they have inherent latency with data transmission which may result in increased time to complete a task, potentially altering clinical assessment. When comparing a baseline assessment to a post-injury assessment, care must be taken to replicate the testing environment as closely as possible to reduce potential confounding variables. C3Logix and two newer ImPACT products, ImPACT quick test and ImPACT pediatric, utilize tablet-based hardware.

Key Points
- Neurocognitive testing is a well-established valuable tool and can be useful to assess for dysfunction in a unique domain not evaluated with other tests.
- Computerized neurocognitive tests are evolving and have their own strengths and limitations; it is important to recognize the strengths and weaknesses of the testing system you are using.
- Neurocognitive testing is meant to be one part of a comprehensive, multimodal concussion evaluation protocol but should not serve as the sole determinant for diagnosis or return to play decisions.
- Consistency of testing is paramount to achieving accurate and repeatable results. Factors affecting testing include testing environment, elimination of distractors, sleep duration and quality, medication usage, and emotional state.

References

1. Randolph C, McCrea M, Barr WB. Is neuropsychological testing useful in the management of sport-related concussion? J Athl Train. 2005;40(3):139–52.
2. Harvey P. Clinical applications of neuropsychological assessment. Dialogues Clin Neurosci. 2012;14(1):91–9.
3. Arrieux J, et al. A review of the validity of computerized neurocognitive assessment tools in mild traumatic brain injury assessment. Future Med Concussion. 2107;2(1)
4. Patricios JS, Schneider KJ, Dvorak J, et al. Consensus statement on concussion in sport: the 6th International Conference on Concussion in Sport-Amsterdam, October 2022. Br J Sports Med. 2023;57(11):695–711. https://doi.org/10.1136/bjsports-2023-106898.

5. Patricios JS, Schneider KJ, et al. Beyond acute concussion assessment to office management: a systematic review informing the development of a Sport Concussion Office Assessment Tool (SCOAT6) for adults and children. Br J Sports Med. 2023;57:737–48. https://doi.org/10.1136/bjsports-2023-106897.
6. O'Connell B, Kelly ÁM, Mockler D, et al. Use of blood biomarkers in the assessment of sports-related concussion-a systematic review in the context of their biological significance. Clin J Sport Med. 2018;28(6):561–71. https://doi.org/10.1097/JSM.0000000000000478.
7. Mann L. On the trail of process: a historical perspective on cognitive process and their training. New York: Grune & Stratton; 1979.
8. Casaletto KB, Heaton RK. Neuropsychological assessment: past and future. J Int Neuropsychol Soc. 2017;23(9-10):778–90. https://doi.org/10.1017/S1355617717001060.
9. McCroy P, et al. Consensus statement on concussion in sport – the 5th international conference on concussion in sport held in Berlin October 2016. Br J Sports Med. 2018;51:838–47.
10. McCroy P, et al. Consensus statement on concussion in sport: the 4th international conference on concussion in sport, Zurich, November 2012. Br J Sports Med. 2013;47:250–8.
11. Bauer R, et al. Computerized neuropsychological assessment devices: joint position paper of the American Academy of Clinical Neuropsychology and the National Academy of Neuropsychology. Arch Clin Neuropsychol. 2012;27(3):362–73.
12. Lindsay DN, et al. Prospective, heat-to-head study of three computerized neurocognitive assessment tools (CNTs): reliability and validity for the assessment of sport-related concussion. J Int Neuropsychol Soc. 2016;22(1):24–37.
13. Roebuck-Spencer T, et al. Assessing change with the Automated Neuropsychological Assessment Metrics (ANAM): issues and challenges. Arch Clin Neuopsychol. 2007;22(Suppl 1):S79–87.
14. Nelson LD, Furger RE, Gikas P, et al. Prospective, Head-to-Head Study of Three Computerized Neurocognitive Assessment Tools Part 2: Utility for Assessment of Mild Traumatic Brain Injury in Emergency Department Patients. J Int Neuropsychol Soc. 2017;23(4):293–303. https://doi.org/10.1017/S1355617717000157.
15. Arrieux JP, Cole WR, Ahrens AP. A review of the validity of computerized neurocognitive assessment tools in mild traumatic brain injury assessment. Concussion. 2017;2(1):CNC31. https://doi.org/10.2217/cnc-2016-0021.
16. Broglio SP, Register-Mihalik JK, Guskiewicz KM, Leddy JJ, Merriman A, Valovich McLeod TC. National athletic trainers' association bridge statement: management of sport-related concussion. J Athl Train. 2024;59(3):225–42. https://doi.org/10.4085/1062-6050-0046.22.
17. Higgins K, et al. Sandbagging on the immediate post-concussion assessment and cognitive testing (ImPACT) in a high school athlete population. Arch Clin Neuropsychol. 2017;32:259–66.
18. Erdal K. Neuropsychological testing for sports-related concussion: how athletes can sandbag their baseline testing without detection. Arch Clin Neuropsychol. 2012;27:473–9.
19. Schatz P, et al. "Sandbagging" baseline test performance on ImPACT, without detection, is more difficult than it appears. Arch Clin Neuropsychol. 2013;28:236–44.
20. Covassin T, et al. Immediate post-concussion assessment and cognitive testing (ImPACT) practices of sports medicine professionals. J Athl Train. 2009;44(6):639–44.

Chapter 7
Concussion Diagnostic Imaging Options

Mani Singh, Jennifer Kordell, and Morteza Khodaee

Clinical Case

A 15-year-old football linebacker collided with another player and has some mild nausea and a headache. After appropriate sideline evaluation, diagnosis of concussion is likely. His parent asks if a diagnostic imaging test should also be performed to aid in diagnosis?

As discussed in the previous chapters, sports-related concussion is largely a clinical diagnosis. In general, the various national and international sports-related concussion guidelines do not recommend routine diagnostic imaging for concussion diagnosis [1–4]. However, as with all medicine, evaluation needs to be individualized and tailored to the specific clinical case. In the remainder of this chapter, we will review when consideration should be given to additional diagnostic imaging and which type may be appropriate in a given clinical scenario.

M. Singh
Sports Medicine Fellow, University of Colorado School of Medicine, Aurora, CO, USA

Department of Rehabilitation and Regenerative Medicine, Columbia University Vagelos College of Physicians and Surgeons, New York, NY, USA

J. Kordell
Family Medicine Resident, University of Colorado School of Medicine, Aurora, CO, USA

M. Khodaee (✉)
Department of Family Medicine and Orthopedics, University of Colorado School of Medicine, Aurora, CO, USA
e-mail: MORTEZA.KHODAEE@CUANSCHUTZ.EDU

© The Author(s), under exclusive license to Springer Nature Switzerland AG 2025
D. S. Patel (ed.), *Concussion Management for Primary Care*,
https://doi.org/10.1007/978-3-031-85516-0_7

X-ray and Computed Tomography (CT)

Question: Should X-ray be ordered for suspected concussion?

The use of X-ray for diagnosis of concussion is not indicated. A document released by the Pediatric Mild Traumatic Brain Injury Guideline Workgroup established by the Centers for Disease Control and Prevention (CDC) National Center for Injury Prevention and Control Board of scientific counselors conducted a literature review from January 1, 1990, to July 31, 2015 [3]. The goal of this review was to create a guideline for recommendations on "diagnosis, prognosis, and management of pediatric mild traumatic brain injury (mTBI)" [3]. As part of this review, evidence was evaluated regarding the necessity of skull radiograph for the diagnosis of pediatric mTBI. The results of this literature review concluded that skull radiographs are not recommended to be used in the diagnosis of pediatric mTBI. Furthermore, skull radiographs are not recommended to be used as a screening tool for intracranial injury. These recommendations are based on two studies that examined the use of skull X-ray in pediatric patients after minor head injury. In one of these studies, possible skull fracture was identified in 7.1% of patients after minor head injury; however, skull radiography is not the best evaluation tool for possible skull fracture. Skull radiography successfully identifies skull fracture in children in only 63% of cases and cannot show details needed to diagnose intracranial injury, such as midline shift. Since head computed tomography (CT) will demonstrate both a skull fracture and many acute intracranial abnormalities, head CT is recommended over X-ray if skull fracture or intracranial injury is suspected [3]. X-ray to evaluate for possible facial and cranial fractures is only recommended in rare situations when a clinical facility does not have access to CT imaging and there is none available in close vicinity. In this instance, X-ray should be considered only if it may help with clinical care and does not delay any transportation to a higher level of care. Indications for head CT in mTBI will be discussed at length in the coming text.

According to a consensus statement on concussion in sport released after a meeting of the Concussion in Sport Group (CISG) in 2022, standard imaging (X-ray, CT, magnetic resonance imaging (MRI)) does not reliably illustrate structural abnormalities of the brain after sports-related concussion. Advanced imaging modalities may identify abnormalities through functional, blood flow, or metabolic studies; however, these studies are currently limited to the research setting [4]. This sentiment is corroborated by the most recent position statement on concussion from the American Medical Society for Sports (AMSSM) [2]. In this position statement, it also recommended that most athletes with suspected sports-related concussion do not need neuroimaging. However, if more serious intracranial injury is suspected, advanced neuroimaging such as MRI or CT is recommended. Specifically, CT is recommended in suspected skull fractures or in cases of suspicion for acute intracranial hemorrhage, whereas MRI may be utilized to evaluate subacute symptoms or in cases with atypical, prolonged recovery. Advanced, multimodal MRI technologies are not yet recommended as additional research is required.

Question: How do I decide if a patient with suspected concussion needs a head CT?

The use of CT for diagnosis of concussion is not routinely recommended. According to guidelines released by the American Academy of Neurology (AAN) in 2013, CT imaging should not be used to diagnose sports-related concussion as currently there is no imaging modality that reliably diagnoses concussion [1]. Instead, CT imaging should be used in situations where more serious traumatic brain injury is suspected. These recommendations are echoed in the aforementioned AMSSM and CISG position statements [2, 4]. This recommendation also holds true for mild traumatic brain injury or concussions unrelated to sport. The 2023 American Congress of Rehabilitation Medicine (ACRM) consensus statement on the diagnostic criteria for mild traumatic brain injury recommends that neuroimaging is generally not necessary to diagnosis a mild TBI [5].

There are multiple decision-making tools specifically aimed at helping clinicians decide if CT is needed after minor head trauma including suspected concussion. The three most common decision tools include the Canadian CT Head Rule (CCHR), the New Orleans Criteria (NOC), and the National Emergency X-Radiography Utilization Study (NEXUS)-II (Table 7.1) [6–8]. The Pediatric Emergency Care Applied Research Network (PECARN), the Canadian Assessment of Tomography for Childhood Head Injury (CATCH)/CATCH2 rules, and the Children's Head Injury Algorithm for the Prediction of Important Clinical Events (CHALICE) are additional sets of clinical decision-making rules for CT in traumatic brain injury specifically aimed at pediatric patients [9, 10].

The Canadian CT Head Rule was developed from a prospective cohort study completed in emergency departments of ten large Canadian hospitals [6]. Patients included in this study had blunt head trauma, witnessed loss of consciousness and

Table 7.1 Comparison of the CCHR, NOC, and NEXUS-II criteria [6–8]

	Canadian head CT rules (CCHR)	New Orleans criteria (NOC)	National emergency X-radiography utilization study II (NEXUS-II) rules
Age	≥65 years	≥60 years	≥65 years
Evidence of trauma	Suspected open or depressed skull fracture Signs of basilar skull fracture	Physical evidence of trauma above the clavicles	Evidence of skull significant skull fracture Scalp hematoma
Neurologic assessment	GCS <15 at 2 h after the injury Amnesia of events prior to impact of greater than 30 minutes	Deficits in short-term memory Drug or alcohol intoxication Seizure	Altered level of alertness Abnormal behavior Neurologic deficit
Emesis	Two or more episodes of vomiting	Vomiting	Persistent vomiting
Other	Dangerous mechanism of injury	Headache	Coagulopathy

disorientation, amnesia, an initial emergency physician determination of Glasgow Coma Score (GCS) of ≥13, and injury within 24 h. The outcome measures of this study included the need for neurological intervention and clinically important brain abnormalities on CT imaging. The need for neurological intervention was defined as death secondary to head trauma within 7 days, or need for procedures including craniotomy, elevation of skull fracture, monitoring of the intracranial pressure, or intubation secondary to head injury. Clinically important brain injuries were defined as any acute findings on CT that would typically warrant hospital admission and neurological follow-up. There were 3,121 patients enrolled in this study, and there was a standardized patient assessment completed by staff physicians board-certified in emergency medicine or by residents in emergency medicine residency programs that were supervised. Based on this initial assessment of patients by the physicians as above, decision was made to either obtain CT of the brain or discharge to home with follow-up via structured 14-day telephone follow-up with a registered nurse. Those patients with concerning telephone follow-up evaluation were brought back to the ER for re-evaluation and head CT. Based on the results of this study, decision rules for determining those minor head injuries that are at higher risk for clinically significant brain injury or neurosurgical intervention readily identified on CT were created. Those symptoms that stratify the patient as high risk for neurological intervention include GCS <15 2 h after the injury, suspected open or depressed skull fracture, signs of basilar skull fracture, two or more episodes of vomiting, and age 65 or higher. Those factors leading to risk for clinically significant brain injury seen on CT include amnesia of events prior to impact of greater than 30 minutes, or a dangerous mechanism (i.e., pedestrian struck by a car, ejected car occupant, fall from height >3 feet or 5 stairs). Combined, these seven factors encompass the Canadian CT Head Rule [6]. Since its introduction, the CCHR has been shown to be a highly sensitive screening tool that may predict the presence of abnormal findings on CT imaging [11]. Studies by Reddy et al. (2023, India) and Habte et al. (2023, Ethiopia) have further validated the CCHR in the international setting as a reliable screening tool that can lead to a reduced number of unnecessary CT scans, thus improving healthcare costs [12, 13]. Furthermore, in a 2023 Clinical Policy statement by the American College of Emergency Physician (ACEP), the use of the CCHR received a Level A recommendation as a first-line decision tool to improve head CT utilization in adults with a minor head injury [14].

The New Orleans Criteria (NOC) were developed after completion of a two-phase study from December of 1997 to June of 1999 [7]. In the first phase of the study, patients with minor head injury (defined as loss of consciousness in combination with normal neurologic examination and GCS of 15) underwent prospective evaluation using a questionnaire to determine clinical findings that best predicted the presence of abnormalities on head CT. This questionnaire was created after review of the literature on minor head injuries and included age, presence or lack of headache, vomiting, intoxication with either drugs or alcohol, short-term memory deficits, post-traumatic seizure, history of coagulopathy, and evidence of trauma above the clavicle. Findings considered to be abnormal on CT in this study included acute traumatic intracranial lesions such as subdural, epidural, parenchymal hematoma, subarachnoid hemorrhage, cerebral contusion, or depressed skull fracture. In the second phase of this study, a questionnaire was administered prior to CT assessing for the seven findings found to have predictive value of intracranial injury in the first phase of the study including headache, vomiting, age, drug/alcohol intoxication, deficits in the short-term memory, physical evidence of trauma about the clavicles, and seizure. In this second group of patients, they were separated into two groups that either had one or more of these findings or met none of these classifications. The rates of positive CT scans were again tallied for each group. Of the 909 patients in both phases of this study, 6.7% of those patients meeting one or more of the aforementioned criteria had abnormal findings on CT scan as compared to 0% of patients meeting none of those criteria. Derived from this study are the New Orleans Criteria, suggesting that patients who have one or more of the following should undergo CT to rule out intracranial injury: headache, vomiting, age over 60 years, drug or alcohol intoxication, deficits in short-term memory, physical evidence of trauma above the clavicles, and seizure. These criteria had a sensitivity of 100 percent for identifying patients with positive CT scans in this study. One criticism of the New Orleans criteria is that it includes headache as a criterion for imaging, yet headache is one of the most common symptoms of concussion. Therefore, many patients with concussions will unnecessarily undergo CT based on these criteria.

The National Emergency X-Radiography Utilization Study (NEXUS)-II is another trial aimed at creating an algorithm for deciding which patients with blunt head trauma should have a head CT [8]. This was a multicenter, prospective, observational study involving 21 hospitals with a total of 13,728 patients. Clinicians decided whether or not to order CT based on clinical judgment rather than a study protocol. Any patient with acute blunt head trauma was enrolled if a CT was ordered for them, and demographic information was obtained for each of these patients in addition to a GCS score. The degree of "neurologic deficit" was recorded for each patient based on a combination of GCS score, presence or absence of motor deficit, abnormal gait, abnormal cerebellar function, and cranial nerve abnormality. If any of these issues were present, the patient was considered to have a neurologic deficit. From this study, eight criteria were identified that were highly associated with intracranial injuries including evidence of significant skull fracture, scalp hematoma, neurologic deficit, altered level of alertness, abnormal behavior, coagulopathy, persistent vomiting, and age 65 years or older. Based on these criteria, 901 of the 917 patients enrolled in this study were identified correctly.

To compare the three aforementioned CT rules for head trauma (CCHR, NOC, and NEXUS-II), a study was done by Ro et al. for the Traumatic Brain Injury Research Network of Korea from 2008–2009 [15]. This study was a prospective, multicenter, observational cohort study of patients with blunt head trauma. Patients were assessed using a standardized protocol in the emergency departments where this study was conducted, and then decision to image with CT was based on clinical judgment of the examining attending physician or resident rather than being dictated by the study protocol. Essentially, each of the study designs for the CCHR, NOC, and NEXUS-II were replicated with the patient population in this study.

Inclusion and exclusion criteria similar to those from each of the three original studies were used, and similar demographic and injury information were obtained as well. There were a total of 7,131 patients that presented with blunt head trauma in this study, with 9.2% of patients meeting CCHR inclusion criteria, 9.8% meeting the NOC inclusion criteria, and 41.4% of patients meeting the NEXUS-II inclusion criteria. The conclusions of this comparison study were that the sensitivities of all three clinical decision-making tools are lower than reported in the original publications; however, the specificities of these three tools are similar to those figures reported in the individual studies. Notably, the CCHR and NOC criteria did not miss any patients requiring neurosurgical intervention. Although, the NEXUS-II criteria decreased the rate of head CT use but also did miss some cases of clinically significant events requiring intervention. The CCHR criteria had a sensitivity of 100% for the five high risk factors identified in the study with a specificity of 68.7% and a positive predictive value (PPV) of 4.37% with negative predictive value (NPV) of 100% [6]. With all seven of the CCHR criteria taken together, their sensitivity for identifying clinically important brain injury was 98.4%, and specificity was 49.6%, while the PPV was 14.7%, and NPV was 99.7% [6]. Regarding the NOC, the sensitivity was found to be 100% and specificity was 25%. The NPV was 100%, while the PPV was 8.2%. The NEXUS-II criteria had a sensitivity of 98.3%, a specificity of 13.7%, and PPV of 50% with NPV of 99.1% [7]. Table 7.2 offers a comparison of the sensitivities, specificities, positive predictive values, and negative predictive values of each of these three decision-making tools.

Similar values were reported in a 2020 systematic review and meta-analysis comparing the CCHR and the NOC [11]. In this study, 14 studies with a total of 21,140 subjects were included for analysis. This study concluded that both the CCHR and NOC were strong tools that could accurately predict the presence of abnormal CT scan findings as well as identifying patients with clinical important TBI (Table 7.3). Both tools were found to have similar sensitivities and positive predictive values. Given this similarity, the authors concluded that the tools might be used interchangeably in special circumstances where contraindications to a specific tool might apply. For example, in the CCHR study, patients were excluded from the study if they were younger than 16 years old, had a bleeding disorder or used oral anticoagulants, or were pregnant [6]. Thus, in these specific populations, the NOC may be applied rather than the CCHR [11].

Table 7.2 Comparing the sensitivities, specificities, positive predictive values, and negative predictive values of the Canadian Head CT rules (CCHR), New Orleans Criteria (NOC), and the National Emergency X-Radiography Utilization Study II criteria [6–8]

	Sensitivity (%)	Specificity (%)	Positive predictive value (PPV) (%)	Negative predictive value (NPV) (%)
CCHR	98.4	49.6	14.7	99.7
NOC	100	25	8.2	100
NEXUS-II	98.3	13.7	50	99.1

Note that the reported values for the CCHR are for all of the seven previously discussed risk factors taken together for prediction of clinically important brain injury

Table 7.3 Comparing the sensitivities, specificities, and diagnostic odds ratio (DOR) of the Canadian Head CT Rules (CCHR) and New Orleans Criteria (NOC) in predicting positive CT findings and identifying clinically important TBI (ciTBI) based on a 2020 systematic review and meta-analysis (95% confidence intervals) [11]

	Sensitivity (%)	Specificity (%)	Diagnostic odds ratio
Prediction of positive CT findings			
CCHR	89.9	38.3	5.5
NOC	97.2	12.3	4.8
Prediction of clinically important TBI			
CCHR	92.5	40.1	8.3
NOC	98.3	8.5	5.4

The accuracy of these three predictive tools were again highlighted in a systematic review done in 2015 by Easter et al. [16]. The authors of this study performed a search of MedLine and the Cochrane library from 1966 to 2015 to find studies dealing with diagnosis of intracranial injuries. There were 14 studies that met inclusion criteria with a total of 23,079 patients. In assessing the accuracy of CCHR, NOC, and NEXUS-II in predicting those patients that are at low risk for significant intracranial injury, it was found that in the absence of meeting any criteria of the CCHR, the probability of severe intracranial injury was 0.31%. In the absence of meeting any criteria of the NOC, the probability of severe intracranial injury was 0.61%, and without any positive criteria from the NEXUS-II criteria, this probability was 3.5% [16].

Question: Are there also CT decision-making rules for children with a head injury?

The Pediatric Emergency Care Applied Research Network (PECARN) group conducted a prospective, cohort study of pediatric patients from 2004 to 2006 to develop guidelines for CT imaging in acute, suspected TBI specifically in children [9]. This study enrolled patients under 18 years of age with head trauma in 25 emergency departments that were part of the PECARN group across the USA. The patient had to be within 24 h of the traumatic event, and the outcomes assessed in this study were death from TBI, need for neurosurgery, intubation greater than 24 h, and hospital admission for greater than or equal to 2 nights (defined as a clinically important TBI). There were a total of 43,904 patients ultimately enrolled in this study. Emerging from this study were seven predictors of more serious injury in pediatric patients including age younger than 2 years, vomiting, loss of consciousness, severe mechanism of injury, severe or worsening headache, amnesia, nonfrontal scalp hematoma GCS score < 15, and clinical suspicion for skull fracture.

The Canadian Assessment of Tomography for Childhood Head Injury (CATCH) rules were presented after a study was done by Osmond et al. published in 2010 [10]. This was a prospective, cohort study carried out in ten Canadian pediatric emergency departments, with patients 0–16 years of age enrolled in this study presenting with minor head injuries. There were a total of 3866 patients participating in this study. There were four high-risk factors and three medium-risk factors that were identified for intracranial injury. The high-risk factors were those that put patients at increased risk for need for neurologic intervention, and the medium-risk factors placed the patient at higher risk for brain injury on CT. The four high-risk factors include "failure to reach GCS of 15 within 2 h of injury, suspicion of open skull fracture, worsening headache, and irritability." The three medium-risk factors identified were "large scalp hematoma, signs of basilar skull fracture, or a dangerous mechanism of injury." Those mechanisms that were deemed dangerous included injuries sustained in a motor vehicle crash, a fall from greater than or equal to 3 feet or five stairs, and a fall from a bike without a helmet. It was found that those high-risk factors identified above had a 100% sensitivity for predicting the need for neurologic intervention with a specificity of 70.2%. A patient having any of the four high-risk factors above, or any of the three medium-risk factors, had a sensitivity of 98.1% for identifying CT evidence of brain injury with a specificity of 50.1% [10].

In 2018, Osmond et al. published an update to their CATCH rules referred to as the CATCH2 rules [17]. This was a multicenter, prospective, cohort study with a total of 4060 enrolled patients. The original seven-item CATCH rule had a sensitivity of 91.3% and 97.5% for predicting the need for neurosurgical intervention and predicting brain injury, respectively. The authors found that adding an 8th criteria, $\geq$ 4 episodes of vomiting, increased these sensitivities to 100% and 99.5%, respectively.

The Children's Head Injury Algorithm for the Prediction of Important Clinical Events (CHALICE) study group performed a prospective, multicenter diagnostic cohort study in order to devise clinical rules that would aid in the identification of high-risk children with head injuries that may require CT scanning [18]. This study recruited 22,772 patients across 10 hospitals in northwestern England between February 2000 and August 2002 under 16 years of age who presented to emergency departments for a head injury without specific other inclusion criteria. The primary outcome measurement was identifying "clinically significant intracranial injury" which were defined as "death as a result of head injury, requirement for neurosurgical intervention, or marked abnormalities on the computed tomography scan." The authors identified 14 specific criteria based on the history, physical examination, and mechanism of injury that would suggest the need for advanced imaging with CT scan – these criteria are listed in Table 7.4 [18]. The study group identified the CHALICE rules as having a 98% sensitivity with an 87% specificity for the prediction of clinically significant head injury.

Table 7.4 provides a helpful overview of the PECARN, CATCH, CATCH2, and CHALICE criteria, while Table 7.5 compares the sensitivities and specificities of the decision rules.

Prior to the formation of the CATCH2 rules, a prospective, cohort study done by Easter et al. in 2015 compared the diagnostic accuracy of the PECARN,CATCH, and CHALICE clinical decision-making rules in diagnosing traumatic brain injury in children. This study was carried out at a Denver hospital and enrolled children younger than 18. There were 1009 patients ultimately included in this study. The three clinical rules were compared regarding the ability to identify clinically important TBI. PECARN had a sensitivity of 100% with a specificity of 62% and a

Table 7.4 The PECARN, CATCH, CATCH2, and CHALICE clinical decision-making rules [9, 10, 17, 18]

PECARN (2009)	CATCH (2010)	CATCH2 (2018)	CHALICE (2006)
<2 years of age Vomiting Loss of consciousness Severe mechanism of injury Severe/worsening headache Amnesia Non-frontal-scalp hematoma GCS<15 Clinical suspicion for skull fracture	Failure to reach GCS of 15 within 2 h of injury (H) Suspected open or depressed skull fracture (H) Worsening headache (H) Irritability (H) Large scalp hematoma (M) Signs of basilar skull fracture (M) Dangerous mechanism of injury (M)	Failure to reach GCS of 15 within 2 h of injury Suspected open or depressed skull fracture Worsening headache Irritability Large scalp hematoma Signs of basilar skull fracture Dangerous mechanism of injury ≥ 4 episodes of vomiting*	Witnessed loss of consciousness (> 5 min duration) Amnesia (>5 min duration) Abnormal drowsiness ≥ 3 episodes of vomiting Suspicion of non-accidental injury Seizure after injury in patient with no history of epilepsy GCS<14 or GCS<15 in children younger than 1 year Suspicion of penetrating or depressed skull injury Signs of basilar skull fracture Positive focal neurologic exam Bruise, swelling, or laceration > 5 cm if < 1 year old High-speed injury (>40 m/h) Fall > 3 m in height High-speed projectile injury

H indicates those factors that place a patient at higher risk for need for neurologic intervention, while M denotes those at "medium risk" who will likely have a traumatic finding on brain CT. When utilizing the CATCH2 rules, any one of these findings suggests the need for head CT. Asterisk indicates new addition from CATCH rules

positive likelihood ratio of 2.7. The CATCH decision rules had a sensitivity of 91%, with a specificity of 44%, and a positive likelihood ratio of 1.6. The CHALICE rules had a sensitivity of 84% with a specificity of 85% and a positive likelihood ratio of 5.5. For those injuries requiring neurosurgical intervention, PECARN had a sensitivity of 100%, with a specificity of 61% and a likelihood ratio of 2.6. CATCH had a sensitivity of 75% with specificity of 43% and a likelihood ratio of 1.3. Finally, CHALICE had a sensitivity of 75%, specificity of 84%, and a likelihood ratio of 4.5 [19].

A more recent retrospective study by Kwon et al. (2021) compared the efficacy of the PECARN and CATCH2 decision rules. The authors determined the sensitivity, specificity, and negative predictive value of the PECARN rules for detecting intracranial pathology to be 80.00%, 28.39%, and 98.58%, respectively. In contrast, the CATCH2 rules were found to have a sensitivity, specificity, and negative predictive value of 100%, 15.25%, and 100%, respectively. Given the higher sensitivity and higher negative predictive value of the CATCH2 rules, the authors concluded this tool to be more appropriate for use in the emergency room setting. One specific limitation of this study is its relatively small sample size (251 patients). Furthermore, caution should be used when interpreting direct comparisons between the PECARN

Table 7.5 Comparing the CATCH, CATCH2, PECARN, and CHALICE clinical decision-making tools regarding their reported sensitivity and specificity

	Sensitivity (%)	Specificity (%)
Need for neurosurgical intervention		
CATCH	91.3	57.1
CATCH2	100	45.7
Findings of brain injury on CT		
CATCH	97.5	59.6
CATCH2	99.5	47.8
Clinically important TBI		
PECARN	96.8[a]–100[b]	53.7[a]–59.8[b]
CHALICE	98	87

CATCH and CATCH2 sensitivities and specificities based on primary outcomes of need for neurologic intervention and findings of brain injury on CT. PECARN sensitivities and specificities reported from validation group in the study for identifying clinically important TBI
[a]Those older than 2 years old in validation groups. CHALICE sensitivities and specificities are based on primary outcome measures of requirement for neurosurgical intervention or marked abnormalities on brain CT
[b]Those less than 2 years old

and CATCH2 rules as the PECARN rules were developed to identify children with low risk of ciTBI (clinically important TBI as defined by any death from TBI, need for neurosurgery, intubation duration greater than 24 h, and hospital admission for greater than or equal to 2 nights) that should not undergo CT scanning, whereas the CATCH2 rules were developed to identify children at high risk of brain injury who should undergo CT scan [20]. In summary, and in accordance with the National Institutes for Health and Care Excellence (NICE) recommendations for investigation of clinically important brain injuries, non-contrast CT is the test of choice for detecting clinically important intracranial injuries given its shorter examination time requirements and ability to reveal neurosurgical emergencies [21]. The decision on whether or not to obtain CT in those patients with head trauma can be guided by the use of one or more of the aforementioned clinical decision tools in addition to general clinical judgment [22].

Magnetic Resonance Imaging (MRI) and Magnetic Resonance Angiography (MRA)

Question: Is an MRI or MRA helpful for diagnosis of concussion?

In acute evaluation of suspected concussion or mTBI, MRI is not recommended based on multiple guidelines [1–4]. According to previously mentioned CDC guidelines on diagnosis and management of mild traumatic brain injury among children, MRI should not be routinely obtained in patients with acute symptoms of mTBI [3]. These sentiments are echoed in recommendations from the AMSSM position statement on concussion in sport [2]. MRI should be reserved for patients with recalcitrant symptoms or for those with suspected underlying chronic brain pathology. Most MRIs done for mTBI fail to reveal any pathology or demonstrate findings that may not be clinically significant such as petechiae or white matter shearing injury [23]. Additionally, a publication from the American Society of Radiologic Technologists (ASRT) on neuroimaging of sports concussions points out that while MRI is better at detecting small lesions in TBI, the amount of time needed in the acute setting to complete the test especially in an emergent setting is unacceptable [24].

There is little evidence to suggest use of magnetic resonance angiography (MRA) in acute concussion. If there are findings concerning for vascular injury on non-contrast CT, either contrast computed tomographic angiography (CTA) or MRA (depending on acuity) should be obtained. MRA is helpful in further elucidating the definition of the vascular walls, whereas CTA is subject to fewer flow artifacts than MRA and also offers better resolution [23].

Other Imaging Modalities

Question: Are there other imaging modalities I should consider obtaining to help diagnose concussion?

There are many imaging modalities currently being developed aimed at detecting the microstructural and microenvironmental brain changes that can occur with concussions including: diffusion tensor imaging (DTI), susceptibility-weighted imaging (SWI), functional MRI (fMRI), arterial spin labeling (ASL), single-photon emission tomography (SPECT) and positron emission tomography (PET), and magnetic resonance spectroscopy (MRS). However, none of these modalities have yet been validated or recommended for current use in a clinical setting for concussion diagnosis or monitoring.

Diffusion Tensor Imaging (DTI)

Diffusion tensor imaging, or DTI, is an MRI method of measuring the diffusion of water across brain tissue. It often measured as fractional anisotropy (FA) which describes the diffusion direction, mean diffusivity (MD) which describes the diffusion magnitude in all directions, axial diffusivity (AD) which describes the diffusion across the main axis and can be an indicator of axonal integrity, and radial diffusivity (RD) which describes the diffusion perpendicular to the main axis and can be an indicator of myelin sheath integrity [25]. FA is usually measured on a scale from 0 to 1 with 0 being diffusion in all directions and 1 being diffusion in a single main axis. Changes in FA, MD, AD, and RD have been reported after mTBI in both the acute and chronic settings, but the change directions have been variable. Some studies demonstrate reduced FA during the acute injury phase which may be a result of axonal swelling or edema; however, other studies report decreased FA and increased MD, RD, and AD 1–2 days after sports-related concussions possibly representing axonal or myelin sheath damage [26–28]. Standards for the use of DTI are still being developed, and current studies have been limited. It is unclear how these changes may be related to clinical symptoms, recovery, and outcomes as these values have been noted to still be changed from baselines 2 months post-injury despite clinical recovery [26]. However, many feel this is a still promising imaging modality for detecting mTBI in the future.

Susceptibility-Weighted Imaging (SWI)

Susceptibility-weighted imaging, or SWI, is another MRI method that is sensitive to hemosiderin and blood products and therefore may be a promising method for detecting microhemorrhages associated with mTBIs. SWI can be analyzed by counting microhemorrhages, hypodensity burden, or isometric magnetic tissue susceptibility [25]. Studies on hockey athletes have shown increased hypodensity burden 2 weeks after a mTBI [29]. Other studies on American football athletes after sports-related concussions showed increased white matter susceptibility. Increased white matter susceptibility on SWI was also associated with longer return-to-play protocols, and as opposed to DTI imaging, these changes correlated to clinical recovery and were no longer present when the athlete recovered and fully returned to play [30]. This is a promising modality for detecting and treating mTBIs given evidence demonstrating a chronological change that correlated to clinical outcomes; however, it is thought to be less sensitive than other methods discussed in this section given its lack of ability to detect the diffuse axonal injury that is believed to be associated with concussions.

Functional MRI (fMRI)

Functional MRI works by assessing cerebral blood flow variations with more active brain tissues requiring more blood flow [25]. It can be used to monitor areas of brain activation during specific tasks (task-based fMRI) or at rest (resting-state fMRI). Increased fMRI signals have been observed in athletes after sports-related concussions during cognitive demand testing in comparison to healthy subjects [31]. Hyperactivation of the specific brain cortices has also been shown to correlate with severity of clinical mTBI symptoms during memory testing [32]. This method may be sensitive to the currently difficult to detect cognitive function changes associated with mTBIs. Resting state fMRIs have also demonstrated increased brain connectivity 1–2 days post-concussion and decreased connectivity and connection strength 5 to 7 and 10 days post-concussion [33, 34]. This method however is very susceptible to environmental and situational changes during testing that may impact the observed cerebral connections. Something as simple as a noise or different visual stimuli during testing may alter the observed fMRI pathways. Additional studies are needed to further assess its use as a clinical diagnostic tool for concussions.

Arterial Spin Labeling (ASL)

Arterial spin labeling, or ASL, is a noninvasive MRI method that measures arterial blood flow to the brain by using magnetically labeled arterial blood water protons as a tracer [25]. Studies have shown reduced cerebral blood flow in the first 24–28 h post-concussion compared to healthy controls [35]. Another study showed blood flow recovery to baseline 1 month post-injury and poorer clinical outcomes with those demonstrating continued reduced cerebral blood flow [36]. However, other studies have struggled to replicate the same clinical correlation and have shown reduced cerebral blood flow despite clinical recovery [37]. Additional studies are needed to investigate the reliability of ASL as a diagnostic tool and for predicting clinical recovery from concussions.

Single-Photon Emission Tomography (SPECT) and Positron Emission Tomography (PET)

Both single-photon emission tomography (SPECT) and positron emission tomography (PET) are functional invasive imaging modalities. SPECT uses radiotracers that are swallowed, inhaled, or injected to indicate where blood flow is in the brain. Brain injury is inferred by decreased blood flow similar to noninvasive ASL methods above. PET uses radiotracers to indicate areas of binding or substance uptake in the brain. Currently novel radiolabeled ligands for PET scans are being developed in hopes of detecting multimodal metabolic changes associated with mTBIs [38]. However, studies on these have been small and inconsistent, and none are yet validated for clinical use. Both SPECT and PET produce images that are of poorer resolution compared to images generated by CT or MRI, and these tests are quite expensive, involve radiation, and are not widely available. For these reasons and others, SPECT and PET are not recommended for use in sports-related mTBI.

Magnetic Resonance Spectroscopy (MRS)

Magnetic resonance spectroscopy (MRS) is a metabolic imaging technique that uses cerebral chemical shift information to combine neurochemical information with neuroanatomy. Using the standard clinical strength of MRI, this method can typically detect the following substances in neural tissue: lactate, N-acetyl-aspartate

(NAA), choline (Cho), myoinositol (mI), and glutamate (Glu), glutamine (Gln), and creatine (Cr). Cr is typically used as an internal reference with the other metabolites being reported as ratios with a Cr denominator. Studies however have been inconsistent as far as increased or decreased levels of these metabolites especially when assessing repeated mTBIs or concussions [25]. Decreased NAA, NAA/Cr ratio, and Glu/Cr ratio have been reported in various anatomical brain locations after a sports-related concussion; however, increased NAA/Cr levels were noted after multiple concussions [34, 39, 40]. Increased mI levels have also been reported 1-month post-concussion [41]. Therefore, single-use MRS does not currently appear to be helpful for sport mTBI diagnosis in the clinical setting, and additional studies investigating longitudinal changes and standardization would be helpful to further clarify the role of MRS in the clinical assessment of sport mTBI in the future.

Key Points
- Diagnostic imaging is not routinely recommended for use in concussion.
- If there is concern for another diagnosis, such as skull fracture or intracranial hemorrhage, a CT scan may be indicated.
- There are multiple decision guidelines available to determine the need for a head CT in adults (CCHR, NOC, and NEXUS-II) and children (PECARN and CATCH2).
- Other diagnostic imaging modalities such as DTI, fMRI, PET, SPECT, and MRS are still being investigated to determine what, if any, clinical role they may play in the diagnosis of concussion.

References

1. Giza CC, Kutcher JS, Ashwal S, Barth J, Getchius TSD, Gioia GA, et al. Summary of evidence-based guideline update: evaluation and management of concussion in sports: report of the Guideline Development Subcommittee of the American Academy of Neurology. Neurology. 2013;80(24):2250–7.
2. Harmon KG, Clugston JR, Dec K, Hainline B, Herring S, Kane SF, et al. American medical society for sports medicine position statement on concussion in sport. Br J Sports Med. 2019;53(4):213–25.
3. Lumba-Brown A, Yeates KO, Sarmiento K, Breiding MJ, Haegerich TM, Gioia GA, et al. Centers for disease control and prevention guideline on the diagnosis and management of mild traumatic brain injury among children. JAMA Pediatr. 2018;172(11):e182853.
4. Patricios JS, Schneider KJ, Dvorak J, Ahmed OH, Blauwet C, Cantu RC, et al. Consensus statement on concussion in sport: the 6th International Conference on Concussion in Sport–Amsterdam, October 2022. Br J Sports Med. 2023;57(11):695–711.
5. Silverberg ND, Iverson GL, ACRM Brain Injury Special Interest Group Mild TBI Task Force Members, et al. The American congress of rehabilitation medicine diagnostic criteria for mild traumatic brain injury. Arch Phys Med Rehabil. 2023;104(8):1343–55.
6. Stiell IG, Wells GA, Vandemheen K, Clement C, Lesiuk H, Laupacis A, et al. The Canadian CT head rule for patients with minor head injury. Lancet. 2001;357(9266):1391–6.
7. Haydel MJ, Preston CA, Mills TJ, Samuel L, Erick B, DeBlieux PMC. Indications for computed tomography in patients with minor head injury. N Engl J Med. 2000;343(2):100–5.

8. Mower WR, Hoffman JR, Herbert M, Wolfson AB, Pollack CV, Zucker MI, et al. Developing a decision instrument to guide computed tomographic imaging of blunt head injury patients. J Trauma. 2005;59(4):954–9.

9. Kuppermann N, Holmes JF, Dayan PS, Hoyle JD, Atabaki SM, Holubkov R, et al. Identification of children at very low risk of clinically-important brain injuries after head trauma: a prospective cohort study. The Lancet. 2009;374(9696):1160–70.

10. Osmond MH, Klassen TP, Wells GA, Correll R, Jarvis A, Joubert G, et al. CATCH: a clinical decision rule for the use of computed tomography in children with minor head injury. CMAJ. 2010;182(4):341–8.

11. Alzuhairy AKA. Accuracy of Canadian CT head rule and New Orleans criteria for minor head trauma; a systematic review and meta-analysis. Arch Acad Emerg Med. 2020;8(1):e79.

12. Reddy A, Poonthottathil F, Jonnakuti R, Thomas R. Efficacy of the Canadian CT head rule in patients presenting to the emergency department with minor head injury. Indian J Crit Care Med. 2024;28(2):148–51.

13. Habte YW, Pajer HB, Abicho TB, Feleke Y, Bizuneh YA, Shao B, et al. Validation of the Canadian CT head rule and the New orleans criteria for mild traumatic brain injury in Ethiopia. World Neurosurg. 2023;173:e600–5.

14. Valente JH, Anderson JD, Paolo WF, Sarmiento K, Tomaszewski CA, Haukoos JS, et al. Clinical policy: critical issues in the management of adult patients presenting to the emergency department with mild traumatic brain injury. Ann Emerg Med. 2023;81(5):e63–105.

15. Ro YS, Shin SD, Holmes JF, Song KJ, Park JO, Cho JS, et al. Comparison of clinical performance of cranial computed tomography rules in patients with minor head injury: a multicenter prospective study. Acad Emerg Med. 2011;18(6):597–604.

16. Easter JS, Haukoos JS, Meehan WP, Novack V, Edlow JA. will neuroimaging reveal a severe intracranial injury in this adult with minor head trauma? The rational clinical examination systematic review. JAMA. 2015;314(24):2672–81.

17. Osmond MH, Klassen TP, Wells GA, Davidson J, Correll R, Boutis K, et al. Validation and refinement of a clinical decision rule for the use of computed tomography in children with minor head injury in the emergency department. CMAJ. 2018;190(27):E816–22.

18. Dunning J, Daly JP, Lomas JP, Lecky F, Batchelor J, Mackway-Jones K, et al. Derivation of the children's head injury algorithm for the prediction of important clinical events decision rule for head injury in children. Arch Dis Child. 2006;91(11):885–91.

19. Easter JS, Bakes K, Dhaliwal J, Miller M, Caruso E, Haukoos JS. Comparison of PECARN, CATCH, and CHALICE rules for children with minor head injury: a prospective cohort study. Ann Emerg Med. 2014;64(2):145–52.

20. Kwon BS, Song HJ, Lee JH. External validation and comparison of the pediatric emergency care applied research network and canadian assessment of tomography for childhood head injury 2 clinical decision rules in children with minor blunt head trauma. Clin Exp Emerg Med. 2021;8(3):182–91.

21. Davis T, Ings A. National Institute of health and care excellence. Head injury: triage, assessment, investigation and early management of head injury in children, young people and adults (NICE guideline CG 176). Arch Dis Child Educ Pract Ed. 2015;100(2):97–100.

22. Lyttle MD, Crowe L, Oakley E, Dunning J, Babl FE. Comparing CATCH, CHALICE and PECARN clinical decision rules for paediatric head injuries. Emerg Med J. 2012;29(10):785–94.

23. Lee B, Newberg A. Neuroimaging in traumatic brain imaging. NeuroRx. 2005;2(2):372–83.

24. Odle TG. Neuroimaging of sports concussions. Radiol Technol. 2017;88(6):621CT–42CT.

25. Esopenko C, Sollmann N, Bonke EM, Wiegand TLT, Heinen F, de Souza NL, et al. Current and emerging techniques in neuroimaging of sport-related concussion. J Clin Neurophysiol. 2023;40(5):398–407.

26. Cubon VA, Murugavel M, Holmes KW, Dettwiler A. Preliminary evidence from a prospective DTI study suggests a posterior-to-anterior pattern of recovery in college athletes with sports-related concussion. Brain Behav. 2018;8(12):e01165.

27. Wu YC, Harezlak J, Elsaid NMH, Lin Z, Wen Q, Mustafi SM, et al. Longitudinal white-matter abnormalities in sports-related concussion: A diffusion MRI study. Neurology. 2020;95(7):e781–92.
28. Mustafi SM, Harezlak J, Koch KM, Nencka AS, Meier TB, West JD, et al. Acute white-matter abnormalities in sports-related concussion: a diffusion tensor imaging study from the NCAA-DoD CARE consortium. J Neurotrauma. 2018;35(22):2653–64.
29. Helmer KG, Pasternak O, Fredman E, Preciado RI, Koerte IK, Sasaki T, et al. Hockey concussion education project, part 1. Susceptibility-weighted imaging study in male and female ice hockey players over a single season. J Neurosurg. 2014;120(4):864–72.
30. Koch KM, Meier TB, Karr R, Nencka AS, Muftuler LT, McCrea M. Quantitative susceptibility mapping after sports-related concussion. AJNR Am J Neuroradiol. 2018;39(7):1215–21.
31. Dettwiler A, Murugavel M, Putukian M, Cubon V, Furtado J, Osherson D. Persistent differences in patterns of brain activation after sports-related concussion: a longitudinal functional magnetic resonance imaging study. J Neurotrauma. 2014;31(2):180–8.
32. Pardini JE, Pardini DA, Becker JT, Dunfee KL, Eddy WF, Lovell MR, et al. Postconcussive symptoms are associated with compensatory cortical recruitment during a working memory task. Neurosurgery. 2010;67(4):1020–7.
33. Churchill NW, Hutchison MG, Richards D, Leung G, Graham SJ, Schweizer TA. The first week after concussion: blood flow, brain function and white matter microstructure. Neuroimage Clin. 2017;14:480–9.
34. Johnson B, Zhang K, Gay M, Horovitz S, Hallett M, Sebastianelli W, et al. Alteration of brain default network in subacute phase of injury in concussed individuals: resting-state fMRI study. Neuroimage. 2012;59(1):511–8.
35. Wang Y, Nencka AS, Meier TB, Guskiewicz K, Mihalik JP, Alison Brooks M, et al. Cerebral blood flow in acute concussion: preliminary ASL findings from the NCAA-DoD CARE consortium. Brain Imaging Behav. 2019;13(5):1375–85.
36. Meier TB, Bellgowan PSF, Singh R, Kuplicki R, Polanski DW, Mayer AR. Recovery of cerebral blood flow following sports-related concussion. JAMA Neurol. 2015;72(5):530–8.
37. Churchill NW, Hutchison MG, Graham SJ, Schweizer TA. Symptom correlates of cerebral blood flow following acute concussion. Neuroimage Clin. 2017;16:234–9.
38. Huang CX, Li YH, Lu W, Huang SH, Li MJ, Xiao LZ, et al. Positron emission tomography imaging for the assessment of mild traumatic brain injury and chronic traumatic encephalopathy: recent advances in radiotracers. Neural Regen Res. 2022;17(1):74–81.
39. Vagnozzi R, Signoretti S, Tavazzi B, Floris R, Ludovici A, Marziali S, et al. Temporal window of metabolic brain vulnerability to concussion: a pilot 1H-magnetic resonance spectroscopic study in concussed athletes – part III. Neurosurgery. 2008;62(6):1286–95.
40. Vagnozzi R, Signoretti S, Cristofori L, Alessandrini F, Floris R, Isgrò E, et al. Assessment of metabolic brain damage and recovery following mild traumatic brain injury: a multicentre, proton magnetic resonance spectroscopic study in concussed patients. Brain. 2010;133(11):3232–42.
41. Churchill NW, Hutchison MG, Graham SJ, Schweizer TA. Neurometabolites and sport-related concussion: from acute injury to one year after medical clearance. Neuroimage Clin. 2020;27:102258.

Chapter 8
Concussion Grading and Prognostic Factors

Raul A. Rosario-Concepcion, Rafael A. Romeu-Mejia,
Robert D. Pagan-Rosado, and Jennifer Roth Maynard

Case

A 15-year-old female with a past medical history of untreated anxiety and a single concussion with protracted recovery earlier this season is brought to your office after getting hit on the back of the head by a volleyball during a serve on practice 2 days ago. The athletic trainer suspected a concussion without loss of consciousness (LOC) and took her off the court for sideline evaluation. Her immediate post-concussion symptom score (PCSS) was elevated, mostly complaining of significant headache, dizziness, and nausea.

What defines prolonged recovery after a concussion?

The most recent International Consensus Statement on Concussion in Sport reports full recovery of symptoms following sports-related concussions (SRC) typically occurs approximately 10–14 days after injury [1] and within 1 month in children aged 0–18 years [2]. Delayed recovery occurs when symptoms persist beyond these expected time frames. Current literature trends suggest using the term

R. A. Rosario-Concepcion (✉)
Department of Physical Medicine and Rehabilitation, Baptist Health South Florida, Miami, FL, USA
e-mail: raul.rosario@baptisthealth.net

R. A. Romeu-Mejia
Department of Physical Medicine and Rehabilitation, Rancho los Amigos National, Rehabilitation Hospital, Downey, CA, USA

R. D. Pagan-Rosado
Department of Physical Medicine and Rehabilitation, Mayo Clinic College of Medicine, Jacksonville, FL, USA

J. R. Maynard
Department of Family Medicine, Mayo Clinic College of Medicine, Jacksonville, FL, USA

D. S. Patel (ed.), *Concussion Management for Primary Care*,
https://doi.org/10.1007/978-3-031-85516-0_8

persistent post-concussive symptoms (PPCS) (i.e., in the physical, cognitive, sleep, and mood domains) following SRC to reflect the failure of normal clinical recovery [1]. Research has increasingly focused on determining which risk factors increase the likelihood of PPCS. Nonetheless, concussion literature regarding recovery time is complex, mixed, and difficult to interpret definitively, whereas each recovery is unique and will follow its own trajectory [3].

Do medical providers still use a concussion grading system to identify severity and prognosis?

In the late 1990s, multiple concussion grading systems were created to classify concussion severity in the attempt to predict outcomes and to help guide return-to-play protocols. These grading systems included the Colorado Medical Society Guidelines, the American Academy of Neurology (AAN) guidelines, and the Cantu guidelines [4, 5]. They incorporated a timeframe and symptomatological variation of LOC, post-traumatic amnesia (PTA), and post-concussion signs/symptoms. The importance of LOC and PTA as reliable markers of severity has been questioned, and recent evidence has failed to correlate the grading systems with injury severity and has not been found to be a reliable predictor of recovery time [6, 7]. These grading systems are no longer used among concussion providers nor recommended by position statements. Current guidelines recommend using different prognostic factors such as age, sex, and past history, among others, to help predict clinical recovery [3, 8].

Should clinicians screen for prognostic factors?

Screening for the presence of prognostic risk factors (Table 8.1) is recommended to initiate earlier intervention and/or appropriate referrals. Both the American Medical Society for Sports Medicine (AMSSM) consensus guideline for SRC and

Table 8.1 Risk factors that may predispose to a prolonged recovery

Age <18
Female gender
Symptom burden (multiple symptoms)
History of mental health disorders
Past history of concussion
Severe on-field signs and symptoms
Past history of migraines
Post-traumatic headaches (especially delayed onset or persistent)
Prolonged rest >5 days
History of learning disability and attention deficit disorder:
Cervical spine dysfunction
Vestibular and oculomotor dysfunction
Delayed reporting or "playing through it"
History of substance abuse
Suboptimal heart rate threshold on BCTT
Completed fewer post-injury assessment time points

the most recent CDC guidelines for pediatric concussion recommend screening for potential risk factors that may contribute to prolonged recovery [3, 8]. These will be discussed in further detail later in this chapter.

In the case above, which are the patient's risk factors that may predispose her to a prolonged recovery?

Age <18

Age is one of the most studied factors related to outcomes after SRC. The few available studies directly examining age-related differences in SRC risk and recovery have produced inconsistent results [9]. Yet, there is some evidence for an age-gradient and level-of-play association with clinical recovery. Overall, trends show faster recovery in professional athletes, followed by college athletes and then high school (HS) athletes [6, 10]. Moreover, a large prospective multicenter study suggested that the teenage and high school years might represent a more vulnerable stage for slow recovery than those of primary school age [11]. However, literature documenting differences in SRC recovery outcomes among adolescents and adults is limited. More research in this area is needed to establish a stronger correlation.

Female Sex

The literature on sex differences regarding recovery time and persistent symptoms is mixed. Overall evidence supports that females take longer to recover, are more likely to have prolonged symptoms, and have greater neurocognitive impairment that their male counterparts [11–14]. Multiple sex-determined differences have been compared and may account for this overall trend. These include differences in neck strength, injury biomechanics, and injury rates in females, as well as higher pre- and post-injury symptom reporting [15]. Ongoing basic science and clinical research may help solidify these underlying differences [16].

Symptom Burden

In an adult cohort with concussion, initial symptom burden (i.e., higher PCSS at first clinical visit within 2 weeks of injury) was more predictive of a SRC recovery >28 days than age, sex, concussion history, and migraine/headache history [17]. This agrees with most studies to date, which consistently show that the strongest predictor of slower recovery from concussion is greater symptom severity following injury both immediately and in the first few days following the injury [1, 6].

History of Mental Health Disorders

Behavioral problems after a concussion are very common and may include depression and anxiety. There is some evidence that pre-injury mental health problems [18], particularly depression and anxiety, have been associated with persistent symptoms after a concussion [11, 19]. Short-term elevated anxiety levels and new-onset anxiety disorders are four times more likely after a mild TBI than after an orthopedic injury [20]. A threefold risk of depression in an adolescent cohort after concussion has also been reported [21]. Prolonged rest or activity restriction has been well described to contribute to anxiety and depressive symptoms in the general population after injury/illness [22]. This is similar after concussions, highlighting the importance of returning patients to their normal environment and activity as soon as medically possible. It is not yet clear, however, whether these are new diagnoses after a concussion or an exacerbation of an underlying predisposition or a subclinical premorbid condition. Referral to a mental health provider for cognitive behavioral therapy should, therefore, be considered when appropriate.

Past History of Concussion

Literature is mixed with regard to associating prior concussion history with clinical outcomes. Whereas some studies have not shown correlation with prolonged recovery [23–25], large-scale retrospective analyses show a link between concussion history and increased risk for symptoms lasting more than 4 weeks [11, 14, 26, 27]. In addition, having a previous concussion with symptoms for ≥ 1 week also correlated with longer recovery in children [11]. Prospective research is needed to strengthen these associations; however, we must certainly consider past concussion history in the clinical setting.

On-Field Signs and Symptoms

Acute signs and symptoms, including presumed injury severity factors, have been greatly scrutinized in literature. While there are mixed findings, most studies have not associated LOC or PTA with recovery [6]. On the other hand, there is some evidence linking presence of retrograde amnesia and slower recovery time, yet a strong relationship has not been demonstrated [6]. A recent systematic review supports that on-field dizziness in children was a consistent predictor for prolonged recovery [28]. Other physical symptoms including nausea, fogginess, and balance, have also been associated with prolonged recovery in very few studies [9]. Overall, literature studying individual symptom association with outcome is limited.

What other prognostic factors are associated with prolonged recovery after concussions?

Past History of Migraines

Pre-injury history of migraine has not been related to outcome in most studies [6]. However, a large, multisite, prospective, well-powered study reported that a pre-injury history of migraine was associated with risk for symptoms lasting more than 4 weeks [11]. More research is needed to definitively establish this association.

Post-traumatic Headaches

Post-traumatic headaches (PTHs) are a common clinical finding in patients who suffered sports-related concussions [9] with approximately 90% of patients experiencing them. Most studies show that acute and subacute PTHs are associated with persistent symptoms [6]. Persistent headaches (>7 days) have been linked to increased recovery time, delayed return to sport, poor cognition, and more symptomatology [9]. It has been reported that PTH with migraine features makes an athlete seven times more prone to recover in >21 days compared to those without these types of headaches [29]. Moreover, the emergence of PTH after 7 days of injury was linked to longer recovery, slow reaction time, reduced memory performance, anterograde amnesia, and an increase in the number of reported symptoms such as nausea, dizziness, and visual changes, among others [9, 30]. More evidence is needed, but all of these factors related to PTH seem to contribute to prolonged recovery and return to play.

Prolonged Rest

Basic science models hypothesize that neurophysiologic disturbances may return to baseline with restriction of neurometabolic demand, i.e., rest. A brief period of 24–48 h of physical and cognitive rest remains the initial step in concussion management [1, 8, 22]. Although immediate removal from the sport and relative rest have shown to be necessary to prevent prolonged recovery [6, 31], a randomized controlled trial of patients aged 11–22 with acute concussion showed that those who underwent strict rest for 5 days vs. usual care (24–48 h. of rest followed by stepwise return to activity) had more daily persistent symptom score and slower recovery [32]. For this reason, strict rest protocols are currently being discouraged [22]. Many studies have reported that extreme withdrawal or "cocooning" patients from daily activities such as school, sports, technology, and the usual pattern of socializing can be linked to psychological issues [8, 33]. Moreover, these issues may translate into poor coping mechanisms which can further lead to increased anxiety and depression—both associated with prolonged recovery time [22]. These maladaptive neuropsychiatric disorders combined with physical deconditioning may exacerbate post-concussive symptoms and delay recovery.

History of Learning Disability and Attention Deficit Disorder

Pediatric patients with a history of learning disabilities have an overall greater life-time concussion incidence [34]. Interestingly, this population has a high prevalence of concussion-like symptoms even in the absence of a concussive injury [35]. Yet, studies have not clearly linked learning disabilities with having more post-concussive symptoms [36]. Nonetheless, in young patients, a history of attention deficit hyper-active disorder (ADHD) has been associated with prolonged recovery from concus-sion [36]. A single-center case-control study involving pediatric patients found that a prior history of ADHD predicted a prolonged recovery (> 28 days) [14]. Another study reported that HS students who sustained a concussion and had pre-injury his-tory of ADHD exhibited a longer, though not statistically significant, time to recov-ery. In this study, the athletes with a pre-injury history of ADHD recovered in 16.5 days compared with the control group who took an average of 13.5 days [37]. In addition, athletes with ADHD can have worsening of ADHD symptoms after a con-cussion [38]. Special consideration is required in order to analyze neurocognitive testing in this population. If the patient is taking a stimulant medication, both base-line and post-concussion testing should be performed after the patient has taken their medication to permit consistent interpretation [38]. More information is needed to strengthen the correlation between ADHD (among other learning dis-abilities) and prolonged recovery.

Cervical Spine Dysfunction

Due to the close proximity of the skull to the cervical spine, the medical provider must consider cervicogenic dysfunction as a possible contributing factor for persis-tent post-concussive symptoms. At the time this chapter was written, there is no standard definition for cervical spine dysfunction (CSD) [39]. One study defines CSD as at least one subjective symptom of cervical spine injury that may include neck pain, headache, or dizziness. In addition, the patient must have some evidence of cervical spine injury during physical examination [39]. Both conditions can have similar mechanism of action and present with nearly similar symptoms [40]. Early findings suggest that CSD may contribute to the development of PPCS, for which more research is needed to establish a stronger correlation [39, 40]. Early intervention with physical rehabilitation including cervical manipulation and muscle strengthening is an important aspect of treatment in this population [40]. Identifying the etiology of certain concussion symptoms from cervicogenic dysfunction source is vital on the evaluation of concussion patients to ensure proper diagnosis and early management.

Vestibular and Oculomotor Dysfunction

Vestibular and oculomotor dysfunctions are the common complaints in the concussed patient. Studies have identified that 81% of concussion patients may develop some form of vestibular dysfunction [41]. Moreover, patients found with vestibular dysfunction or dizziness on initial evaluation tend to take more time to return to school/sports than those without [41–43]. In regard to oculomotor complaints, convergence insufficiency is one of the main causes for eye strain, headaches, and blurred vision [44]. Oculomotor disturbances related to concussion may affect reading, note-taking, and technology use among other daily life activities [41]. More specifically, as seen in a retrospective study, vestibulo-ocular deficits are one of the many risk factors that may extend recovery [45]. Literature has well documented deficient performances on neurocognitive tests among patients with receded near point of convergence (NPC) [46]. Additionally, a recent study reported that patients with convergence insufficiency revealed gait deficits not present in either healthy controls or those without NPC insufficiency [47]. For this reason, early symptom identification with subsequent vestibulo-ocular rehabilitation is important to improve the patient's vestibulo-ocular symptoms and prognosis [48].

Delayed Reporting or "Playing Through It"

Underreporting of concussion symptoms is an issue that can curtail the removal of an athlete from physical activity following concussion [49]. Studies have revealed that between 30% and 50% of concussions go unreported by athletes, displaying a dependence on self-reported symptoms and the need for objective diagnostic measures [49]. A recent study indicated that athletes who were not immediately removed from activity following concussion had a longer recovery and missed more days of activity versus those who were quickly removed from play [31]. Delayed reporting of symptoms was linked to a recovery that lasted 5 days longer than those who immediately reported symptoms [31]. Other related studies have also found that delayed removal from play has been associated with a longer recovery time [6].

Substance Abuse

In many cases, substance abuse may mask the symptoms of mild TBI thus challenging the assessment of risk factors that may alter prognosis [50]. Literature has reported deficits in executive functioning and memory among abusers, as well as poor post-concussive mood stability among patients with a history of abuse. All of these deficits exacerbate post-concussive symptomatology and have been shown to prolong recovery [51, 52]. Moreover, patients who have a history of mood disorders under treatment may exhibit chronic alterations of brain structures that regulate emotions caused by long-term substance (i.e., medication) use. These alterations along with post-injury substance abuse also curtail concussion rehabilitation [52, 53].

Heart Rate Threshold

The Buffalo Concussion Treadmill Test (BCTT) is a validated analysis that allows measuring the amount of aerobic exercise that is safe to perform following concussion. It is based on the maximum heart rate (termed heart-rate threshold [HRt]) achieved when exacerbation of symptoms occur [54]. In a randomized controlled trial in acutely concussed adolescents, a HRt of <135 bpm during BCTT was associated with a recovery of >21 days [55, 56]. This cutoff value was only studied in adolescents and may not be useful in other patient populations due to differences in cardiovascular fitness and those with baseline heart rate variability [57]. These variables must be taken into account in order to reach a more standardized cutoff. Moreover, a recent study on concussions patients discussed that a heart-rate change (HRt, baseline HR) of less than 50 bpm was 73% sensitive and 78% specific for predicting prolonged recovery (>30 days) [58]. More prospective studies are needed in this regard to further elucidate these associations.

Is there any evidence for risk factor modification to improve outcomes after concussion?

Although age and gender are not modifiable, early risk factor modification is key in the management of concussion. The correct identification of these prognostic factors can help guide rehabilitation in concussed athletes. *Return-to-activity/play programs need to be individualized for each patient in order to achieve better outcomes.* As described above, there is strong evidence for immediate removal of a person from high-risk contact activity and short-term (48–72 h) rest, followed by symptom-limited activity with the goal of avoiding protracted recovery. Reinforcing these recommendations, a prospective multicenter cohort study by Grool and colleagues showed that children and adolescents who participated in at least light aerobic exercise within 7 days following an acute concussion had a lower risk of PPCS at

Table 8.2 Treatment options for persistent post-concussive symptoms (PPCS)

Early identification of concussion symptoms and screening of risk factors for prolong recovery
Adequate referral and management of previously diagnosed mental health disorders
Appropriate management of past history of migraines or headaches
Avoidance of prolonged strict rest
Referral if needed for evaluation of learning disability and treatment of attention deficit disorder
Physical therapy to address cervical spine, vestibular and/or oculomotor dysfunction
Identification or management of substance abuse
Buffalo Concussion Treadmill Test (BCTT) to develop an early return-to-physical activity program

28 days vs. controls who didn't engage in physical activity [59]. In addition, there is increasing support for use of therapeutic submaximal HRt activity in patients with chronic symptoms or PPCS to facilitate recovery [55, 56, 60]. Overall, growing evidence, current consensus, and clinical experience suggest that gradual return of physical activity should begin as soon as tolerated following concussion while avoiding high-risk activities that could result in another TBI [1, 22].

Each concussive injury is unique in its mechanism, symptomatology, and formulation of modifiers that may impact prognosis. Management should be individualized according to the athlete's presentation (Table 8.2). Clinicians should be aware of their State law and league guidelines for safe return to play.

Key Points

- Concussion grading systems are no longer used in the medical community and clinical practice.
- Screening for the presence of prognostic risk factors is recommended to initiate earlier intervention and/or appropriate referrals.
- Demographic characteristics such as younger age (<18 years old) and female sex may be associated with longer recoveries.
- Past history of concussion, migraines, and psychiatric and learning disabilities (e.g., anxiety, depression, ADHD) may be linked with persistent post-concussive symptoms.
- Individual symptoms have variable associations with longer recovery (e.g., post-traumatic headache, dizziness, fogginess, etc.) as well as cervicogenic and vestibular/oculomotor dysfunction after a concussion.
- Higher initial concussion symptom scores (i.e., symptom burden) has the strongest association with prolonged recovery.
- While prolonged rest for >5 days has negative correlation with recovery, early progression of physical activity within the first week (guided by the symptom exacerbation threshold) shows an inverse relationship.
- Return-to-activity/play programs need to be individualized for each patient in order to achieve better outcomes.

References

1. Patricios JS, Schneider KJ, Dvorak J, et al. Consensus statement on concussion in sport: the 6th international conference on concussion in sport–Amsterdam, October 2022. Br J Sports Med. 2023;57:695–711.
2. Barlow KM, Crawford S, Stevenson A, Sandhu SS, Belanger F, Dewey D. Epidemiology of postconcussion syndrome in pediatric mild traumatic brain injury. Pediatrics. 2010;126(2):e374–81. https://doi.org/10.1542/peds.2009-092574.
3. Lumba-Brown A, Yeates K, Sarmiento K, et al. Centers for disease control and prevention guideline on the diagnosis and management of mild traumatic brain injury among children. JAMA Pediatr. 2018;172(11):e182853. https://doi.org/10.1001/jamapediatrics.2018.2853.
4. Cantu RC. Posttraumatic retrograde and anterograde amnesia: pathophysiology and implications in grading and safe return to play. J Athl Train. 2001;36:244–8.
5. Quality Standards Subcommittee. Report of the quality standards subcommittee. Practice parameter: the management of concussion in sports (summary statement). Neurology. 1997;48:581–5.
6. Iverson GL, Gardner AJ, Terry DP, Ponsford JL, Sills AK, Broshek DK, Solomon GS. Predictors of clinical recovery from concussion: a systematic review. Br J Sports Med. 2017;51(12):941–8.
7. Makdissi M, Darby D, Maruff P, Ugoni A, Brukner P, McCrory P. Natural history of concussion in sport. Am J Sports Med. 2010;38(3):464–71. https://doi.org/10.1177/0363546509349491.
8. Harmon KG, Clugston JR, Dec K, et al. American medical society for sports medicine position statement on concussion in sport. Br J Sports Med. 2019;53:213–25.
9. Elbin RJ, D'Amico N, McLeod TV, Covassin T, Anderson M. Concussion: predicting recovery. In: Musahl V, Karlsson J, Krutsch W, Mandelbaum B, Espregueira-Mendes J, d'Hooghe P, editors. Return to play in football. Berlin, Heidelberg: Springer; 2018. https://doi.org/10.1007/978-3-662-55713-6_54.
10. Covassin T, Elbin RJ, Harris W, Parker T, Kontos AP. The role of age and sex in symptoms, neurocog- nitive performance, and postural stability in athletes after concussion. Am J Sports Med. 2012;40(6):1303–12.
11. Zemek R, Barrowman N, Freedman SB, et al. Clinical risk score for persistent postconcussion symptoms among children with acute concussion in the ED. JAMA. 2016;315:1014–25.
12. Kostyun R, Hafeez I. Protracted recovery from a concussion a focus on gender and treatment interventions in an adolescent population. Sports Health. 2015;7(1):52–7.
13. Bock S, Grim R, Barron TF, et al. Factors associated with delayed recovery in Athletes with concussion treated at a pediatric neurology concussion clinic. Childs Nerv Syst. 2015;31:2111–6.
14. Miller JH, Gill C, Kuhn EN, Rocque BG, Menendez JY, O'Neill JA, et al. Predictors of delayed recovery following pediatric sports related concussion: a case-control study. J Neurosurg Pediatr. 2016;17:491–6. https://doi.org/10.3171/2015.8.PEDS14332.
15. Brown DA, Elsass JA, Miller AJ, et al. Differences in symptom reporting between males and females at baseline and after a sports-related concussion: a systematic review and meta-analysis. Sports Med. 2015;45:1027–40.
16. Giza C, Greco T, Prins ML. Handbook of clinical neurology, vol. 158. Elsevier B.V.; 2018. p. 51–61.
17. Meehan WP III, O'Brien MJ, Geminiani E, Mannix R. Initial symptom burden predicts duration of symptoms after concussion. J Sci Med Sport. 2016;19(9):722–5.
18. Morgan CD, Zuckerman SL, Lee YM, et al. Predictors of postconcussion syndrome after sports-related concussion in young Athletes: a matched case-control study. J Neurosurg Pediatr. 2015;15:589–98.
19. Eisenberg MA, Andrea J, Meehan W, et al. Time interval between concussions and symptom duration. Pediatrics. 2013;132:8–17.

20. Luis CA, Mittenberg W. Mood and anxiety disorders following pediatric traumatic brain injury: a prospective study. J Clin Exp Neuropsychol. 2002;24(3):270–9. https://doi.org/10.1076/jcen.24.3.270.982.
21. Chrisman SP, Richardson LP. Prevalence of diagnosed depression in adolescents with history of concussion. J Adolesc Health. 2014;54(5):582–6.
22. DiFazio M, Silverberg ND, Kirkwood MW, Bernier R, Iverson GL. Prolonged activity restriction after concussion. Clin Pediatr. 2015;55(5):443–51. https://doi.org/10.1177/0009922815589914.
23. Ellis MJ, Ritchie LJ, Koltek M, et al. Psychiatric outcomes after pediatric sports-related concussion. J Neurosurg Pediatr. 2015;16:709–18.
24. McCrea M, Guskiewicz K, Randolph C, et al. Incidence, clinical course, and predictors of prolonged recovery time following sport-related concussion in high school and college Athletes. J Int Neuropsychol Soc. 2013;19:22–33.
25. Barlow M, Schlabach D, Peiffer J, et al. Differences in change scores and the predictive validity of three commonly used measures following concussion in the middle school and high school aged population. Int J Sports Phys Ther. 2011;6:150–7.
26. Corwin DJ, Zonfrillo MR, Master CL, et al. Characteristics of prolonged concussion recovery in a pediatric subspecialty referral population. J Pediatr. 2014;165:1207–15.
27. Guskiewicz KM, et al. The NCAA concussion study. J Am Med Assoc. 2003;290:2549–55.
28. Davis GA, Anderson V, Babl FE, Gioia GA, Giza CC, Meehan W, Moser RS, Purcell L, Schatz P, Schneider KJ, Takagi M, Yeates KO, Zemek R. What is the difference in concussion management in children as compared with adults? A systematic review. Br J Sports Med Published Online First. 2017;28 https://doi.org/10.1136/bjsports-2016-097415.
29. Kontos AP, Elbin RJ, Lau B, Simensky S, Freund B, French J, Collins MW. Posttraumatic migraine as a predictor of recovery and cognitive impairment after sport-related concussion. Am J Sports Med. 2013;41(7):1497–504. https://doi.org/10.1177/0363546513488751.
30. Collins MW, Field M, Lovell MR, et al. Relationship between post concussion headache and neuropsychological test performance in high school athletes. Am J Sports Med. 2003;31:168–73. https://doi.org/10.1177/03635465030310020301.
31. Asken BM, McCrea MA, Clugston JR, Snyder AR, Houck ZM, Bauer RM. "Playing through it": delayed reporting and removal from athletic activity after concussion predicts prolonged recovery. J Athl Train. 2016;51(4):329–35. https://doi.org/10.4085/1062-6050-51.5.02.
32. Thomas DG, Apps JN, Hoffmann RG, et al. Benefits of strict rest after acute concussion: a randomized controlled trial. Pediatrics. 2015;135:213–23.
33. Edmed S, Sullivan K. Depression, anxiety, and stress as predictors of post concussion-like symptoms in a non-clinical sample. Psychiatry Res. 2012;200:41–5. https://doi.org/10.1016/j.psychres.2012.05.022.
34. Iverson GL, Wojtowicz M, Brooks BL, Maxwell BA, Atkins JE, Zafonte R, et al. High school athletes with ADHD and learning difficulties have a greater lifetime concussion history. J Atten Disord. 2016; https://doi.org/10.1177/1087054716657410.
35. Iverson GL, Atkins JE, Zafonte R, et al. Concussion history in adolescent athletes with attention-deficit hyperactivity disorder. J Neurotrauma. 2016;33:2077–80. https://doi.org/10.1136/bjsports-2017-097729.
36. Zuckerman SL et al. Prognostic factors in pediatric sport-related concussion. Current Neurology and Neuroscience Reports. U.S. National Library of Medicine. 2018. https://doi.org/10.1007/s11910-018-0909-4.
37. Mautner K, Sussman WI, Axtman M, Al-Farsi Y, Al-Adawi S. Relationship of attention deficit hyperactivity disorder and postconcussion recovery in youth athletes. Clin J Sport Med. 2015;25:355–60. https://doi.org/10.1097/JSM.0000000000000151.
38. Pujalte GGA, Maynard JR, Thurston MJ, Taylor WC, Chauhan M. Considerations in the care of athletes with attention deficit hyperactivity disorder. Clin J Sport Med. 2017;1 https://doi.org/10.1097/jsm.0000000000000508.

39. Ellis M, McDonald P, Olson A, Koenig J, Russell K. Cervical spine dysfunction following pediatric sports-related head trauma. J Head Trauma Rehabil. 2019;34(2):103–10. https://doi.org/10.1097/htr.0000000000000411.
40. Cheever K, Kawata K, Tierney R, Galgon A. Cervical injury assessments for concussion evaluation: a review. J Athl Train. 2016;51(12):1037–44. https://doi.org/10.4085/1062-6050-51.12.15.
41. Corwin D, Wiebe D, Zonfrillo M, et al. Vestibular deficits following youth concussion. J Pediatr. 2015;166(5):1221–5. https://doi.org/10.1016/j.jpeds.2015.01.039.
42. Ellis M, Leddy J, Willer B. Physiological, vestibulo-ocular and cervicogenic post-concussion disorders: an evidence-based classification system with directions for treatment. Brain Inj. 2014;29(2):238–48. https://doi.org/10.3109/02699052.2014.965207.
43. Chorney S, Suryadevara A, Nicholas B. Audiovestibular symptoms as predictors of prolonged sports-related concussion among NCAA athletes. Laryngoscope. 2017;127(12):2850–3. https://doi.org/10.1002/lary.26564.
44. Lavrich JB. Convergence insufficiency and its current treatment. Curr Opin Ophthalmol. 2010;21:356–60. https://doi.org/10.1097/ICU.0b013e32833cf03a.
45. Ellis MJ, Cordingley D, Vis S, et al. Vestibulo-ocular dysfunction in pediatric sports-related concussion. J Neurosurg Pediatr. 2015;16:248–55. https://doi.org/10.3171/2015.1.PEDS14524.
46. Pearce KL, Sufrinko A, Lau BC, et al. Near point of convergence after a sport-related concussion: measurement reliability and relationship to neurocognitive impairment and symptoms. Am J Sports Med. 2015;43:3055–61. https://doi.org/10.1177/0363546515606430.
47. Howell DR, et al. Near point of convergence and gait deficits in adolescents after sport-related concussion. Clin J Sport Med. 2018;28(3):262–7. https://doi.org/10.1097/jsm.0000000000000439.
48. Broglio S, Collins M, Williams R, Mucha A, Kontos A. Current and emerging rehabilitation for concussion. Clin Sports Med. 2015;34(2):213–31. https://doi.org/10.1016/j.csm.2014.12.005.
49. Meehan WP, Mannix RC, O'Brien MJ, Collins MW. The prevalence of undiagnosed concussions in athletes. Clin J Sport Med. 2013;23(5):339–42. https://doi.org/10.1097/JSM.0b013e318291d3b3.
50. Allen DN, Goldstein G, Caponigro JM, Donohue B. The effects of alcoholism comorbidity on neurocognitive function following traumatic brain injury. Appl Neuropsychol. 2009;16:186–92. https://doi.org/10.1080/0908428090309868.
51. Conner KR, Pinquart M, Gamble SA. Meta-analysis of depression and substance use among individuals with alcohol use disorders. J Subst Abuse Treat. 2009;37:127–37. https://doi.org/10.1016/j.jsat.2008.11.007.
52. Unsworth D, Mathias J. Traumatic brain injury and alcohol/substance abuse: a Bayesian meta-analysis comparing the outcomes of people with and without a history of abuse. J Clin Exp Neuropsychol. 2017;39:547–62. https://doi.org/10.1080/13803395.2016.1248812.
53. Oscar-Berman M, Marinković K. Alcohol: effects on neurobehavioral functions and the brain. Neuropsychol Rev. 2007;17:239–57. https://doi.org/10.1007/s11065-007-9038-6.
54. Leddy JJ, Willer B. Use of graded exercise testing in concussion and return-to-activity management. Curr Sports Med Rep. 2013;12:370–6. https://doi.org/10.1249/jsr.0000000000000008.
55. Leddy JJ, Haider MN, Ellis M, Willer BS. Exercise is medicine for concussion. Curr Sports Med Rep. 2018;17(8):262–70. https://doi.org/10.1249/jsr.0000000000000505.
56. Leddy JJ, Hinds AL, Miecznikowski J, Darling S, Matuszak J, Baker JG, et al. Safety and prognostic utility of provocative exercise testing in acutely concussed adolescents: a randomized trial. Clin J Sport Med. 2018;28:13–20. https://doi.org/10.1097/JSM.0000000000000431.
57. Sarganas G, Rosario AS, Neuhauser HK. Resting heart rate percentiles and associated factors in children and adolescents. J. Pediatr. 2017;187(174–81):e3. https://doi.org/10.1016/j.jpeds.2017.05.021.

58. Haider MN, Leddy JJ, Wilber CG, Viera KB, Bezherano I, Wilkins KJ, Miecznikowski JC, Willer BS. The predictive capacity of the buffalo concussion treadmill test after sport-related concussion in adolescents. Front. Neurol. 2019;10:395. https://doi.org/10.3389/fneur.2019.00395.
59. Grool AM, Aglipay M, Momoli F, Meehan WP, Freedman SB, et al. Association between early participation in physical activity following acute concussion and persistent postconcussive symptoms in children and adolescents. JAMA. 2016;316(23):2504. https://doi.org/10.1001/jama.2016.17396.
60. Leddy JJ, Kozlowski K, Donnelly JP, Pendergast DR, Epstein LH, Willer B. A preliminary study of subsymptom threshold exercise training for refractory post-concussion syndrome. Clin J Sport Med. 2010;20(1):21–7.

Chapter 9
Concussion Treatment

Nathan Falk, T. Jason Meredith, Jake Herber, and Joshua Bertollo

Clinical Case

A 16-year-old and his mother present to clinic for evaluation of a possible concussion. The patient plays soccer and suffered a head-to-head collision with a teammate the night prior. He did not have any immediate symptoms but began experiencing headache, photophobia, and dizziness after practice. He slept poorly overnight and is very fatigued today. He attended school today but struggled throughout the day with worsening symptoms; the mother wants to know when he can return to school. The patient would like to know if he can play in his game tomorrow night.

The treatment of concussions has historically been based on consensus guidelines, clinical experience, and observational studies. Newer studies have changed how we use exercise in the management of concussion [1–3]. Initial management focuses on preventing patients from suffering another blow to the head by immediately removing them from competition and limiting possible exposures until they are symptom-free. Symptom-limited exercise has been shown to improve the time frame in return-to-baseline status [1–3]. The traditional return to play (RTP) model has been modified to include an active recovery/rehabilitation phase and a RTP phase. The management of concussion requires a great deal of time and patient/caregiver education on the provider's part. General brain health measures such as hydration, adequate sleep, and healthy dietary intake are encouraged as well, as they are often overlooked.

N. Falk (✉) · J. Bertollo
Florida State University, Winter Haven, FL, USA
e-mail: nfalk@fsu.edu; joshua.bertollo@baycare.org

T. J. Meredith · J. Herber
University of Nebraska Medical Center, Omaha, NE, USA
e-mail: jason.meredith@unmc.edu; jacob.herber@unmc.edu

© The Author(s), under exclusive license to Springer Nature
Switzerland AG 2025
D. S. Patel (ed.), *Concussion Management for Primary Care*,
https://doi.org/10.1007/978-3-031-85516-0_9

107

Question: What is the best initial management of sports-related concussion (SRC)?

Previously, strict rest for the first 48 h after concussion was the standard recommendation; however, research now demonstrates that strict rest produces suboptimal outcomes. Recommending strict rest/complete cognitive rest/"cocooning" may increase negative effects on patients in the form of social isolation and psychological distress [1, 4]. Therefore relative (not strict) rest is recommended immediately and for up to the first 48 h after a concussion, which includes activities of daily living (ADL) and reduced/limited screen time [4]. Patients who engage in early high cognitive exertion have shown longer recovery times [5]. Light mental and physical activities are indicated, provided they do not more than mildly exacerbate symptoms. Mild exacerbation of symptoms has been defined as an increase in symptom severity by 2 (on a 1–10 scale) that lasts for more than 1 hour [4].

A more accurate recommendation may be to limit activities that aggravate the patient's particular symptoms, but not put patients at risk for complete social and cognitive isolation. For example, if phonophobia is present, reducing volume on devices and using noise cancelling headphones or ear plugs may be of benefit. If photophobia or bright screens are aggravating, screens can be dimmed, and duration of exposure can be limited. If there are eye-tracking or balance issues, certain content can be limited such as avoiding watching fast action sports and video games while the brain recovers. Light intensity physical activity such as light-paced walking, stationary biking, and household chores that do not more than mildly exacerbate symptoms can be recommended during the first 24–48 h [4]. Healthcare providers are encouraged to recommend and reassure patients and families that light intensity physical activity is safe, with the reminder that activity should not more than mildly exacerbate symptoms [4]. Early light intensity physical activity improves SRC symptoms at a faster rate and decreases the risk for post-concussion symptoms [4–6]. Importantly, risk of contact, collision, or fall when performing light activity must be avoided, which often requires patient and family education.

Screen time guidance should be individualized. Limiting patients to minimal screen time may worsen somatic symptoms compared to symptom-limited moderate screen time [6, 7]. There does not appear to be data to support reduced screen time after the first 48 h; however, the patient should be encouraged to limit screen time based on symptom exacerbation [7]. A joint decision-making process should be incorporated in determining a reasonable screen time allotment while recovering. With children and adolescent patients, it is important to remember the idiom "if you give them an inch, they will take a mile." Providers must emphasize the importance of following symptom-limited screen time. Excess screen time, especially near bedtime, can interfere with sleep quality which is important in concussion recovery. Ultimately, proper patient and family education on gauging symptom severity to guide recovery is imperative to ensure expected recovery timelines.

Question: What is the role of exercise in treating concussions?

Prescribed early exercise treatment plans have been shown to reduce delayed recovery and persistent post-concussive symptoms [1]. The use of early exercise may also shorten the time prior to clearance for RTS [1]. Clinic-based exercise programs (physician or physical therapist offices) may lead to faster recovery and RTP; however, the associated time commitment and logistical concerns such as transportation may limit their feasibility [1]. Home exercise programs can also be safely completed if guidelines that outline exercise intensity and symptom monitoring are closely adhered to. Patients and parents should be educated that advancing too swiftly could cause a prolonged recovery and symptom course [4]. A standardized approach is now freely available for providers to access [4] (https://bjsm.bmj.com/content/57/11/695). Under this approach, stages 1–3 are active recovery/rehabilitation for SRCs utilizing sub-symptom threshold exercise. Once patients are symptom-free and return to the classroom without restrictions, they may progress to stages 4–6 which focus on return to play/sport; each stage should take approximately 24 h. Please see dedicated chapter on Return to Play for further details.

Question: When should a concussed student resume school (return to school)

The transition back to school and learning or return to learn (RTL) is an important consideration, as the goal is returning to "pre-injury learning" without new academic support [4]. Much of those decisions on timing will depend on the patient's current severity of symptoms, limitations or exacerbating factors, and tolerance of academic work. Please see dedicated chapter on Return to Learn for further details.

Most athletes have a complete RTL by day 10 without additional academic support [4, 6]; however, significant variability in this can occur. Certain populations, for example, high-acuity symptom severity or a prior learning disability, may affect the recovery process [4]. Initially, providers should recommend relative rest with the goal of getting the patient back to school in some form within 1–2 days of suffering their concussion. Prolonged school absence can lead to academic disruptions and social isolation [6]. Providers should work with their local schools to maximize their patient's symptom-limited school participation by utilizing various environmental, physical, curricular, and testing accommodations. Options for accommodations include providing alternate school schedules, breaks as needed during the school day, use of hats/sunglasses for photophobia, additional time for assignments and testing, delaying of examinations, use of headphones for noise reduction, limiting screen time with use of paper instead of screen-based resources, and/or avoidance of busy, noisy, or crowded environments [1, 4, 6–8].

Question: The mother proceeds to ask what medications would be safe for him to take for his headache?

Concussions can cause a wide variety of symptoms, but one of the most common and disabling symptoms is headache [8]. By practicing relative mental and physical rest from activities, most symptoms should resolve with time. The current literature on medical management of concussions is lacking, but some medications are used in moderation for patient symptoms. It is important to differentiate whether the headache is more migraine or tension-related. Current treatment of headaches is largely empiric, but more specific therapy can be guided depending on what is causing the headache. In the acute setting, acetaminophen and nonsteroidal anti-inflammatory drugs (NSAIDs) can be used and are considered initial therapy once intracranial bleeding has been excluded [8]. Naproxen is a reasonable choice for moderate-to-severe headache symptoms given its longer half-life [8]. Chronic use of NSAIDs and acetaminophen should be avoided and limited to shortest duration possible [8, 9]. Alternating acetaminophen and ibuprofen may lead to the least amount of post-concussive headache days and best return-to-school rate [8, 9]. For headaches that are not alleviated by simple analgesics and have migraine features, triptans may be a reasonable abortive therapy [10]. For headaches that are more frequent and persistent (for several weeks), preventive medications such as tricyclic antidepressants may be considered [10]. These medications usually are not initiated during the initial acute treatment phase and typically require titration to demonstrate benefit [8]. The delayed onset of benefit should be discussed with the patient and family to avoid false expectations [8]. Tricyclic antidepressants may also be beneficial because they may address post-concussive sleep disturbances and mood disorders [10].

Minimal data currently exists regarding the efficacy of amitriptyline or other preventive medications for persistent post-concussive headache in the pediatric population. Most benefits of preventive medications have been extrapolated from data on migraine management [8]. The side effects of these medications should also be thoroughly explained and discussed with the patient and family. If neck symptoms and tension-related headaches are predominant symptoms, patient education about posture, early neck stretches, and range of motion exercises are important. The use of physical therapy and osteopathic manipulation treatment (OMT) in combination with analgesics for tension-related headaches may be helpful [11, 12]. Physical therapy and OMT may be initiated early in the treatment process and may be particularly beneficial if there is a cervical component to headaches that can frequently occur when there is a whiplash-type mechanism at the time of their concussion injury [11, 12]. Muscle relaxers and antispasmodic medications are rarely used because their side effects often compound other concussive symptoms [6].

Question: What treatments are available to treat dizziness from a concussion?

Dizziness ranks as one of the most common symptoms after a concussion. Most cases resolve within 3 weeks without specific intervention [13]; however, prolonged dizziness often requires a multidisciplinary team. Initially, dizziness should be managed conservatively with education on limiting rapid position changes and head movements [6]. For severe symptoms, off-label meclizine usage has historically been considered as a treatment option, but there is no evidence to support this practice. For many patients the dizziness may episodic and lasting less than a few minutes, which may not allow adequate time for meclizine to take effect.

There are many different causes of dizziness in concussion: benign paroxysmal positional vertigo, balance dysfunction, cervicogenic dizziness, exercise-induced dizziness, visual motion sensitivity, and vestibulo-ocular reflex impairment [13] Providers should consider cervico-vestibular rehabilitation if headache, neck pain, and/or dizziness last for more than 10 days; focused rehabilitation has been shown to be beneficial in symptom reduction and overall recovery [4]. In patients with persistent symptoms of dizziness for more than 3 weeks, benign positional paroxysmal vertigo (BPPV) is the most likely cause [13]. Patients who undergo BPPV positional repositioning can have significant improvement, so providers should be familiar with these techniques or be willing to refer early for proper repositioning/rehabilitation. In patients who continue to suffer from dizziness after 3 months, further evaluation should be performed to rule out central nervous system abnormalities [13].

Question: Is there any medication that can improve the cognitive symptoms of a concussion?

No approved pharmaceutical interventions currently exist for addressing cognitive problems linked to concussions. Many of the hypotheses regarding the efficacy of attention deficit disorder medications in managing concussions are based on information from animal research or human studies involving individuals with more severe traumatic brain injury [14]. Inferring the use of current medications becomes challenging based on the appropriate application, range of symptoms, and brief duration of most moderate brain injuries. Medicine may be warranted in cases where the severity of symptoms significantly impairs one's capacity to engage in academic or occupational activities and/or have persisted for a minimum of 1 month following a concussion. Assessing whether symptoms are being managed due solely due to pharmaceutical masking or measuring true cognitive recovery can be challenging when using additional medications.

Certain medications have been assessed for the treatment of cognitive impairments caused by concussions, although their usage is controversial and their regular use is not recommended. Amantadine has been prescribed to improve cognitive function through induction of the release of dopamine and its NMDA receptor antagonistic properties. Theoretically, this medicine could enhance speed and cognitive efficiency and reduce overall symptoms. Initial research was promising and indicated that the use of amantadine may influence overall functional improvement in post-concussive recovery and enhance neuroprotective properties following an injury. Improvements in reported symptoms of verbal memory and reaction time performance when compared to a control group were also noted [15, 16]. In follow-up studies, amantadine did not improve measurable outcomes of cognitive function [17]. The data surrounding amantadine is conflicting and warrants additional investigation for its potential application in post-concussion recovery [17, 18]. Drugs that impact cognition throughout the post-concussion recovery process are a subject of debate and require careful consideration the potential hazards and benefits for each patient.

Question: Do attention deficit disorder medications have a role in treating attention symptoms of a concussion?

Often, challenges in cognitive processing and lack of focus following a concussion prompt the question of attention deficit drugs as a potential intervention in the management of concussions.

The administration of methylphenidate is considered due to its favorable tolerability and demonstrated efficacy in managing severe brain injury. Although data are promising, it is important for healthcare providers to be aware that methylphenidate has not received FDA approval particularly for the treatment of inattentiveness resulting from concussions. Stimulant use among athletes with ADHD was independently associated with reduced incidence for concussion and lower deviation from baseline in verbal memory, visual memory, and motor skills, post-concussion [19]. Several research articles have reported the additional advantage of utilizing this medicine to enhance concentration and processing speed throughout the recovery [19, 20]. Research has demonstrated that methylphenidate is most effective when administered during the subacute treatment stage of a concussion. Patients who receive stimulant-based medications prior to concussion are advised to continue with their use throughout the recovery period [19].

Question: How does sleep play a role in recovery?

Concussions frequently result in sleep disruption affecting both duration and quality of sleep. Adequate sleep is essential for optimal cognitive recovery post-concussion [21]. Individuals with sleep disturbances within 2 weeks of concussion have been found to have more severe concussion symptoms including dizziness, headaches, and difficulties with emotional regulation in the post-concussive recovery phase [22, 23]. The duration and frequency of daytime sleep or naps should not be so excessive to interrupt a normal circadian rhythm or interrupt the natural sleep cycle. In the acute recovery period, brief naps of 20 min or less in duration may be appropriate.

Sleep education is critical for concussion recovery, emphasizing the importance of addressing sleep disturbances to facilitate optimal recovery outcomes. Sleep quality, duration, and early intervention strategies are key areas of focus in research aimed at improving post-concussion care. Counseling on sleep hygiene, including video screen and blue light avoidance near bedtime, is a critical first step. Consumption of caffeine and alcohol might significantly impact sleep patterns; therefore patients should be educated on limitations and timing of alcohol and caffeine consumption. Alcohol consumption should generally be avoided during the period of concussion recovery not only for sleep but its cognitive impacts as well. Melatonin may be explored as a treatment option when symptoms do not improve and sleep disturbances persist despite receiving appropriate instruction and excellent sleep hygiene. The recommended dosages for melatonin in pediatric and adolescent patients is 3–5 mg. There is limited empirical support to substantiate its efficacy in facilitating long-term healing. Most published research primarily focuses on the utilization of melatonin during the acute phase and have not been extensively examined over an extended period of time [24]. Melatonin prescription was not associated with faster symptom recovery. Research has indicated that trazodone may have advantageous effects; however, its side effect profile and its potential to induce reduced REM sleep in patients limit use. Other sleep aids such as zolpidem are occasionally contemplated for use in the adults but should be avoided in pediatric patients. Caution should be taken when utilizing this medication due to its adverse side effect profile, which mimics the symptoms such as tiredness and cognitive impairment, similar to those seen in the post-concussive state and therefore should be prescribed only as needed on a case-by-case basis. Cognitive-behavioral therapy for insomnia (CBT-I) was shown to reduce sleep disturbances and enhancing recovery outcomes in individuals with persistent post-concussion symptoms [25]. The decreased sleep disturbances were shown to decrease the neuropsychiatric effects of concussion. It is crucial to emphasize the importance of adequate sleep and address sleep disturbances to facilitate optimal recovery.

Question: Are any supplements (fish oil, turmeric, vitamins) recommended to help with recovery?

Data on supplement efficacy is sparse, but adequate nutrition and a multivitamin with C, D, and E, along with omega-3, during the recovery period is reasonable to recommend. Both magnesium and vitamin B6 may be useful for headaches, including migraine and post-traumatic ones [26, 27]. Magnesium supplementation (400 mg once-twice daily) has been shown to improve post-concussion symptoms, including headache. B6 (25–100 mg daily) has been shown to improve headache symptoms and may be useful in nausea management, similar to what is seen in pregnancy.

Omega-3 Fatty Acid

Data suggests that omega-3 fatty acids may have a positive impact on the healing process of major brain injuries; however, there is insufficient evidence about their effectiveness in less severe injuries like concussions. Omega-3 fatty acids are often suggested by practitioners due to their ability to aid in brain recovery. However, there is a lack of human research that provides indications of the additional advantages associated with this supplement [28]. Patients who were supplementing with omega-3 fatty prior to injury showed protection against reduction in plasticity of neurons and subsequent impaired learning via normalization of levels of proteins associated with neuronal circuit function, cognitive processing, synaptic facilitation, neuronal excitability, and locomotor control [29].

Vitamins D and E

In an animal model study, vitamin D at doses of 1 mcg/kg/day was suggestive of decreased neuronal and axonal death in the post-TBI model [30]. Another research model proposed that 2 IU/kg/day of vitamin E improved cognition in following multiple concussions. In addition to increased cognition, vitamin E was shown to lower the oxidative stress in the animal model [31]. In one study, vitamin E was found to reduce mortality and improve long-term functional outcomes after significant TBI, and low serum vitamin E has been associated with poorer prognosis after TBI with intracranial injury [32, 33]. Given the lack of concussion-specific studies, care should be taken in extrapolating these data to concussions. The most reasonable path would be to ensure adequate nutrition and perhaps a multivitamin during recovery.

Turmeric

Turmeric is utilized as a supplement for a variety of conditions due to its anti-inflammatory properties, and animal research has demonstrated diminished brain inflammation after traumatic injury [29]. Curcumin, the active ingredient in turmeric, was found to significantly mitigate the effects of inflammatory markers such as IL-1β, IL-6, and TNF-α and was also shown to reduce the oxidative stress factors levels. The animal models also note that curcumin increases neuron survival rate by increasing the effects of synapsin I, which portends greater neurological function by reducing cerebral edema [34, 35]. In human studies, curcumin doses of 100–3000 mg daily were shown to produce favorable results following TBI [36]. Further research is required to confirm dosing; however, usual supplementary dosing of 500 mg BID-TID seems reasonable to recommend.

Key Points
- While strict physical and cognitive rest for at least the first 48 h post-injury had been the mainstay of recommendations, relative rest and sub-symptom-worsening level activity has been shown to yield superior outcomes to strict rest.
- Early exercise treatment plans have been shown to reduce delayed recovery and persistent post-concussive symptoms.
- Although limited data has been used to support prescribing amantadine and neuro-stimulant medications, no FDA-approved medications currently exist, and their routine use in sports-related concussions is not recommended.
- In patients with ADHD, medications used prior to concussion should be continued during the recovery period.
- While data are somewhat limited, supplementation with vitamins C, D, and E (usually via a multivitamin), omega-3, magnesium, and B6 are all reasonable and may aid in recovery and decrease post-concussion headaches.

References

1. Leddy JJ, Burma JS, Toomey CM, Hayden A, Davis GA, Babl FE, et al. Rest and exercise early after sport-related concussion: a systematic review and meta-analysis. Br J Sports Med. 2023;57(12):762–70.
2. Leddy JJ, Haider MN, Ellis MJ, Mannix R, Darling SR, Freitas MS, et al. Early subthreshold aerobic exercise for sport-related concussion. JAMA Pediatr. 2019;173(4):319.
3. Leddy JJ, Master CL, Mannix R, Wiebe DJ, Grady MF, Meehan WP, et al. Early targeted heart rate aerobic exercise versus placebo stretching for sport-related concussion in adolescents: a randomized controlled trial. Lancet Child Adolescent Health. 2021;5(11):792–9.
4. Patricios JS, Schneider KJ, Dvorak J, Ahmed OH, Blauwet C, Cantu RC, et al. Consensus statement on concussion in sport: the 6th international conference on concussion in sport–Amsterdam, October 2022. Br J Sports Med. 2023;57(11):695–711.
5. Cairncross M, Yeates KO, Tang K, Madigan S, Beauchamp MH, Craig W, et al. Early postinjury screen time and concussion recovery. Pediatrics. 2022;150(5)
6. Putukian M, Purcell L, Schneider KJ, Black AM, Burma JS, Chandran A, et al. Clinical recovery from concussion–return to school and sport: a systematic review and meta-analysis. Br J Sports Med. 2023;57(12):798–809.
7. Macnow T, Curran T, Tolliday C, Martin K, McCarthy M, Ayturk D, et al. Effect of screen time on recovery from concussion: a randomized clinical trial. JAMA Pediatr. 2021;175(11):1124–31.
8. Irwin SL, Kacperski J, Rastogi RG. Pediatric post-traumatic headache and implications for return to sport: a narrative review. Headache J Head Face Pain. 2020;60(6):1076–92.
9. Patterson Gentile C, Shah R, Irwin SL, Greene K, Szperka CL. Acute and chronic management of posttraumatic headache in children: a systematic review. Headache J Head Face Pain. 2021;61(10):1475–92.
10. Pearson R, Levyim D, Choe M, Taraman S, Langdon R. Survey of child neurologists on management of pediatric post-traumatic headache. J Child Neurol. 2019;34(12):739–47.
11. Esterov D, Thomas A, Weiss K. Osteopathic manipulative medicine in the management of headaches associated with postconcussion syndrome. J Osteopath Med. 2021;
12. Quatman-Yates CC, Hunter-Giordano A, Shimamura KK, Landel R, Alsalaheen BA, Hanke TA, et al. Physical therapy evaluation and treatment after concussion/mild traumatic brain injury. J Orthop Sports Phys Ther. 2020;50(4):CPG1–73.
13. Gianoli GJ. Post-concussive dizziness: a review and clinical approach to the patient. Front Neurol. 2022;4:12.
14. Huang CH, Huang CC, Sun CK, Lin GH, Hou WH. Methylphenidate on cognitive improvement in patients with traumatic brain injury: a meta-analysis. Curr Neuropharmacol. 2016;14(3):272–81.
15. Schneider W, Drew-Cates J, Wong T, Dombovy M. Cognitive and behavioural efficacy of amantadine in acute traumatic brain injury: an initial double blind placebo-controlled study. Brain Injury. 1999;13(11):863–72.
16. Meythaler J, Brunner R, Johnson A, Novack T. Amantadine to improve neurorecovery in traumatic brain injury-associated diffuse axonal injury: a pilot double-blind randomized trial. J Head Trauma Rehabil. 2002;17(4):300–13.
17. Hammond F, Sherer M, Malec J, Zafonte R, Dikmen S, Bogner J, Bell K, Barber J, Temkin N. Amantadine did not positively impact cognition in chronic traumatic brain injury: a multisite, randomized, controlled trial. J Neurotrauma. 2018;35(19):2298–305.
18. Loggini A, Tangonan R, Ammar F, Mansour A, Goldenberg F, Kramer C, Lazaridis C. The role of amantadine in cognitive recovery early after traumatic brain injury: a systematic review. Clin Neurol Neurosurg. 2020;194:105815.
19. Ali M, Dreher N, Hannah T, Li A, Asghar N, Spiera Z, Marayati NF, Durbin J, Gometz A, Lovell M, Choudhri T. Concussion incidence and recovery among youth athletes with ADHD taking stimulant-based therapy. Orthop J Sports Med. 2021;9(10):23259671211032564.

20. Rabinowitz A, Watanabe T. Pharmacotherapy for treatment of cognitive and neuropsychiatric symptoms after mTBI. J Head Trauma Rehabil. 2020;35(1):76–83.
21. Fisher M, Wiseman-Hakes C, Obeid J, DeMatteo C. Does sleep quality influence recovery outcomes after postconcussive injury in children and adolescents? J Head Trauma Rehabil. 2023;38(3):240–8.
22. Howell DR, Potter MN, Provance AJ, Wilson PE, Kirkwood MW, Wilson JC. Sleep problems and melatonin prescription after concussion among youth athletes. Clin J Sports Med. 2021;31(6):475–80.
23. Smulligan KL, Wilson JC, Seehusen CN, Wingerson MJ, Magliato SN, Howell DR. Post-concussion dizziness, sleep quality, and postural instability: a cross-sectional investigation. J Athl Train. 2021;57(11–12):1072–8.
24. Barlow K, Brooks B, MacMaster F, Kirton A, Seeger T, Esser M, Crawford S, Nettel-Agirre A, Zemek R, Angelo M, Kirk V, Emery C, Johnson D, Hill M, Buchhalter J, Turley B, Richer L, Platt R, Hutchison J, Dewey D. A double-blind, placebo-controlled intervention trial of 3 and 10 mg sublingual melatonin for post-concussion syndrome in youths (PLAYGAME): study protocol for a randomized controlled trial. Trials. 2014;15(271):1–10.
25. Ludwig R, Rippee M, D'Silva LJ, Radel J, Eakman AM, Morris J, Drerup M, Siengsukon C. Assessing cognitive behavioral therapy for insomnia to improve sleep outcomes in individuals with a concussion: protocol for a delayed randomized controlled trial. JMIR Res Protoc. 2022;11(9):e38608.
26. Standiford L, O'Daniel M, Hysell M, Trigger C. A randomized cohort study of the efficacy of PO magnesium in the treatment of acute concussions in adolescents. Am J Emerg Med. 2021;44:419–22.
27. Nematgorgani S, Razeghi-Jahromi S, Jafari E, Togha M, Rafiee P, Ghorbani Z, Ahmadi Z, Baigi V. B vitamins and their combination could reduce migraine headaches: a randomized double-blind controlled trial. Curr J Neurol. 2022;21(2):105–18.
28. Barrett E, McBurney M, Ciappio E. ω-3 acid supplementation as a potential therapeutic aid for the recovery from mild traumatic brain injury/concussion. Adv Nutr. 2014;5:268–77.
29. Ashbaugh A, McGrew C. The role of nutritional supplements in sports concussion treatment. Head Neck Spine. 2016;15(1):16–9.
30. Tang H, Hua F, Wang J, Yousuf S, Atif F, Sayeed I, et al. Progesterone and vitamin D combination therapy modulates inflammatory response after traumatic brain injury. Brain Injury. 2015;1–10
31. Aiguo W, Zhe Y, Gomez-Pinilla F. Vitamin E protects against oxidative damage and learning disability after mild traumatic brain injury in rats. Neurorehabil Neural Repair. 2010;24(3):290–8.
32. Razmkon A, Sadidi A, Sherafat-Kazemzadeh E, Mehrafshan A, Jamali M, Malekpour B, et al. Administration of vitamin C and vitamin E in severe head injury: a randomized double-blind controlled trial. Clin Neurosurg. 2011;58:133–7.
33. Park G, Ro Y, Yoon H, Lee S, Jung E, Moon S, Kim S, Shin S. Serum vitamin E level and functional prognosis after traumatic brain injury with intracranial injury: a multicenter prospective study. Front Neurol. 2022;13:1008717.
34. Zhu HT, Bian C, Yuan JC, Chu WH, Xiang X, Chen F, Wang CS, Feng H, Lin JK. Curcumin attenuates acute inflammatory injury by inhibiting the TLR4/MyD88/NF-κB signaling pathway in experimental traumatic brain injury. J Neuroinflammation. 2014;27(11):59. https://doi.org/10.1186/1742-2094-11-59.
35. Dong W, Yang B, Wang L, Li B, Guo X, Zhang M, et al. Curcumin plays neuroprotective roles against traumatic brain injury partly via Nrf2 signaling. Toxicol Appl Pharmacol. 2018;346:28–36. https://doi.org/10.1016/j.taap.2018.03.020.
36. United States Patent Bennett et al. US009101580B2 US 9,101,580 B2 Aug. 11, 2015 (10) Patent No.: (45) Date of Patent: (54) Compositions and methods for treating traumatic brain inuryus9101580b2

Chapter 10
Concussion Return to Learn or Work and Return to Play

Suraj Achar and Alec Contag

Clinical Case

You are evaluating a 16-year-old track-and-field athlete for concussion after a fall 2 weeks ago at practice. She denies any loss of consciousness or posttraumatic amnesia. She has been staying home from school after being prescribed strict brain rest by her primary physician, but symptoms have yet to fully resolve. The patient and her mother are asking when it will be safe to leave the house and resume school.

Consensus guidelines endorse 24–48 h of symptom-limited cognitive and physical rest followed by a gradual increase in activity staying below symptom exacerbation thresholds.

The original rational for longer post-injury rest related to both symptom management and faster recovery. Rest was believed to minimize brain energy demands following concussion. Lower energy demand would theoretically lessen post-concussion symptoms and promote recovery. Unfortunately, current evidence is insufficient to prove rest achieves either one of these objectives. To the contrary, a 2015 prospective randomized control trial showed that in post-sports-related concussion (SRC), recommending strict rest for 5 days offered no added benefit over 1–2 days of rest followed by gradual return to activity [1]. The strict rest group reported more daily post-concussive symptoms and had slower symptom resolution [1]. A follow-up multicenter prospective cohort study in 2016 reconfirmed that prolonged rest (avoidance of physical activity for 7 days post-concussion) was

S. Achar (✉)
Department of Family medicine, Department of pediatric orthopedics,
UCSD & Rady Children's hospital, San Diego, CA, USA

A. Contag
Department of Family Medicine, UCSD Sports Medicine Fellow, San Diego, CA, USA

associated with increased incidence of persistent post-concussive symptoms [2]. As of 2023, current recommendations include a brief period of relative rest (24–48 h) during the acute phase after injury, followed by gradual increase in activity while staying below individualized symptom exacerbation thresholds. Relative rest is defined as avoidance of cocooning after the injury, while completing activities of daily living (ADLs), walking, and brief cognitive loads immediately after injury [3]. Healthcare providers (HCPs) with access to exercise testing can safely start patients on sub-symptom threshold aerobic exercise 2–10 days after sports-related concussion (SRC). Aerobic exercises should be tailored to the individual's heart rate threshold (HRt), meaning exercise should stay below the level that causes more than a mild increase in symptoms (a two-point increase on a 0–10 scale). Exercise intensity can be gradually increased by regularly, retesting the HRt and adjusting as needed [4].

Question: Are there risks associated with prolonged rest?

Since 2001, when the Concussion in Sport Group (CISG) released its consensus statement encouraging active rest until asymptomatic, much has changed regarding our approach to managing return to learn (RTL) and return to play in athletes who are recovering from SRC.

There are multiple factors that may contribute to the negative outcomes associated with prolonged rest after concussion. Inactivity contributes to exercise intolerance and physical deconditioning [4]. Missed school and social isolation lead to increased anxiety, depression, and discouragement about recovery. Catastrophizing may also contribute to perpetual symptoms [5–7].

Researchers set out to determine if there were any potential adverse effects of early return to activities in symptomatic patients. Brooks et al. used computerized cognitive testing on adolescents in the emergency department and showed that the early increase in cognitive stress (by way of computerized neurocognitive testing immediately after diagnosis of concussion) did not worsen symptoms at follow-up (7–10 days, 1 month, 2 months, and 3 months). Early cognitive stress also did not prolong symptom recovery compared to the control group [8]. In 2017, Leddy et al. set out to determine if there was any relationship between early physical activity and concussion symptom recovery/duration. Using a prospective randomized control trial, they determined that exercise using the Buffalo Concussion Treadmill Test within 1 week of diagnosis of SRC did not affect recovery. Additionally, they found that the degree of early exercise intolerance after sports-related concussion was an important prognostic factor with implications for academic and team preparation [9].

Question: Are there any advantages of early light aerobic activity?

As research continued to emerge showing that sports-related concussion patients did not seem to have adverse effects with early subthreshold physical activity, Leddy et al. continued to assess the potential positive aspects of early aerobic exercise [10]. In 2019, they published a randomized control trial of concussed adolescents showing that individualized sub-symptom threshold aerobic exercise treatment during the first week after SRC expedited recovery and may reduce the incidence of delayed recovery [10].

Question: When is an athlete fully recovered and how long does it typically take?

The 2016 CISG guidelines state that athletes should return to a baseline level of symptoms, but they do not provide objective definitions to establish when an athlete is fully recovered. As of 2023 no universal definition of full recovery or symptom resolution has been adopted [3]. Resolution of symptoms is critical to recovery but is insufficient on its own. Likewise, symptom reporting alone may be problematic if athletes are underreporting symptoms. Diagnosing symptom resolution can be challenging, as post-concussion-like symptoms may be present in non-concussed individuals, both at rest and during exercise. [11]. Healthy adolescents, for example, have been shown to have symptom severity scores up to 6 (out of a maximal 132) when given a concussion checklist to complete [12]. As such, some studies use a symptom cut off score of less than 7 to define symptom recovery consistent with "baseline level of symptoms" in the 2016 CISG guidelines. Clinical recovery can therefore be defined functionally in Table 10.1.

Most athletes, regardless of age or biological sex, with SRC return to learn by 10 days and to sport by 2–3 weeks [3]; however, studies have shown that complete resolution of physiological/visual and balance function may take up to 3–4 weeks [13]. The latest concussion in sport guidelines has defined persistent post-concussive symptoms, as symptoms lasting greater than 4 weeks in adults and children [4]. Up to 30% of adults and children with SRC can experience persisting post-concussive symptoms based on standardized and validated symptom rating scales [14]. New research suggests that adults and adolescents with greater than 10 days of headache, dizziness, or neck pain, and children with 5 days of dizziness may benefit from cervicovestibular physical therapy to aid in faster recovery [15]. Sleep quality and length have also been frequently implicated as an avenue for delayed recovery, although evidence of the highest quality is still lacking [16].

Table 10.1 Suggested functional definition of concussion recovery. To meet the definition of functional recovery, a concussed person must meet EITHER one Ia or Ib, as well as II and III

	Functional definition of concussion recovery
I	(a) Symptom resolution at rest: No symptoms associated with current concussion at rest
	(a) Complete symptom resolution: No symptoms during/after maximal physical and cognitive exertion
II	Complete return to learn: Return to pre-injury level of school/work without additional supports after a staged return-to-learn strategy
III	Complete return to sport: Return to sport with complete symptom resolution, including return to baseline balance and cognitive functioning after completing a return-to-sport strategy

Question: Are there additional metrics useful for informing return to learn/ play decisions?

Neurocognitive testing has been widely used to assess concussion and track cognitive recovery. A 2010 national survey of concussed high school athletes found that approximately 40% of US high schools that employ an athletic trainer use computerized neurocognitive tests when managing sports-related concussions [17]. Testing is discussed in depth in a separate chapter. We address it briefly here as it is commonly used in return to play decisions (see "Concussion Neurocognitive Testing" chapter).

Neurocognitive tests can provide a more objective measure of brain-behavior relationships and are believed to be important given the potential unreliability of self-reporting symptoms after injury. In a case control study comparing concussed and non-concussed athletes, at 2 days post-injury the addition of neurocognitive testing resulted in an increase in sensitivity of 19%, leading authors to conclude that neurocognitive testing can increase diagnostic accuracy when used in conjunction with self-reported symptoms [18].

In the 2018 American Medical Society for Sports Medicine (AMSSM) position statement on concussion in sport, it was asserted that most concussions can be managed appropriately without the use of neurocognitive testing [19]. According to the AMSSM, when used, neurocognitive testing should be part of a comprehensive concussion management strategy. The statement reiterates that testing should be interpreted by healthcare professionals trained and familiar with the type of test and individual test limitations. It also highlights that comprehensive neurocognitive evaluation can be helpful in management of athletes with persistent symptoms or complicated courses [19]. In our clinic for patients with prolonged concussion, we take a multidisciplinary approach with neurocognitive testing administered and evaluated by a neuropsychologist. We track changes in performance over time with testing providing another data point to help guide our management.

Question: How do you implement return to learn?

To date, evidence shows that SRC can have short-term effects on learning with possible academic dysfunction for up to 1 month [20] but overall minimal impact on long-term academic performance [21]. Most athletes, of any age or sex, returned to learn at 10 days without additional academic supports [3]. For students transitioning back to the classroom, return to learn should be performed in an individualized but stepwise process. In our practice we follow the protocol outlined in Table 10.2. This mirrors the recommendations from the 2022 CISG consensus statement. Immediately post-injury, an initial stage of relative brain rest for 24–48 h is recommended. Students then advance to partial school participation where they attend a few hours of school and only complete necessary assignments, avoid testing and loud areas, and have breaks available as needed. If symptoms are significant and exacerbated at school, students may need to rest in a quiet area versus the nurse's office or leave school for the day and ideally return the next day. As patients tolerate increasing

Table 10.2 Return-to-learn table [3]

Stage	Home activity	School activity	Physical activity	Goal of step
Relative brain rest	Sleep as much as needed (at least 8 h) Allow short naps (<1 h) during day Start transition toward regular sleep/wake cycle Avoid bright light if bothersome Stay well hydrated and eat healthy snacks q3–4 h Limit screen time; use large font	No school No homework May begin easy tasks at home (drawing, baking, cooking) Soft music/audio books Limit screen time as symptoms tolerate during first 48 h (i.e., 10–15 min intervals)	Walking short distances to get around (RTP stage 1) No strenuous exercise or contact sports No driving	Gradual return to typical activities
Rest stage should be limited to 24–48 h post-injury only				
Return to school (partial day)	Strict sleep-wake cycle with goal 8 h of sleep at night Avoid napping during day Stay well hydrated and eat healthy snacks q3–4 h Limit screen time and social activities outside of school as symptoms tolerate	Start with a few hours/half days Sit in front of class Take a break in nurse's office or quiet room q2 hrs only PRN Avoid loud areas (music, band, choir, shop class, locker room, cafeteria loud hallway, and gym) Sunglasses/brimmed hat/ear plugs PRN Preprinted (large font -18) class notes Complete necessary assignments only Limit homework No tests or quizzes Tutoring or note taker as needed Stop work if symptoms increase	No high-intensity physical activity or contact sports (RTP stage 2A) No driving	Increase tolerance to cognitive work

(continued)

Table 10.2 (continued)

Stage	Home activity	School activity	Physical activity	Goal of step
Progress to next stage as symptoms improve and can tolerate activities without increasing symptoms				
Return to school full day	Strict sleep-wake cycle with at least 8 h of sleep at night Avoid napping during day Stay well hydrated and eat healthy snacks q3–4 h Screen time and social activities outside of school as symptoms tolerate	Progress to attending core classes for full days Add in electives when tolerated No more than one test or quiz per day Give extra time or untimed homework/ tests Tutoring or help as needed Stop work if symptoms increase	No high-intensity physical activity or contact sports (RTP stage 2B) OK to drive	Increase academic activities
Progress to next stage when in school full time and completing all assignments without symptoms				
Full recovery	Return-to-normal home and social activities	Return-to-normal school schedule and course load	OK to progress to return to play stage 3	Return to full academic activities and catch up on missed work

demands without symptom exacerbation, they gradually return to a normal course and activity load.

During transition back to the classroom following a concussion, a clear set of academic supports should be provided to allow for early screening, quick intervention, and progress monitoring (Table 10.3). The 2022 Amsterdam consensus statement on concussion in sport notes that RTL is enhanced by environmental physical curriculum and testing adjustments [4].

For the return to learn to be immediate and effective, general education teachers must be trained and empowered to front-load academic supports within the first 4 weeks and should fade academic supports as the concussion symptoms resolve [22]. If these supports are not adequate, then increasing to a more formal intervention in the way of an individualized education plan (IEP) or a 504 plan is warranted. Section 504 of the Rehabilitation Act is a federal civil rights law that provides protection if a person has a physical or mental impairment. A 504 plan may be considered if a medical condition substantially limits at least one of the major life activities (i.e., thinking, concentrating, reading, sleeping, or learning). 504 plans are an ideal mechanism for use in the return-to-learn process for the remaining 30% of patients with symptoms that are severe and or lasting longer than the expected recovery of 4 weeks. However, requesting a 504 plan or IEP too soon following a concussion can delay rapidly needed academic supports for students by diverting time and energy into legal or policy-based processes [22].

Table 10.3 Example of physician-recommended school accommodations following concussion

Area	Physician-requested modifications
Breaks	[] If symptoms worsen during class, allow student to go to quiet area or nurse's office; if no improvement after 30 min, dismissal to home [] Allow breaks during day as deemed necessary by student or teachers/school personnel
Visual stimulus	[] Enlarged print (18 font) copies of textbook material/assignments [] Pre-printed notes (18 font) or note taker for class material [] Limited computer, TV screen, bright screen use [] Allow handwritten assignments (as opposed to typed on a computer) [] Allow student to wear sunglasses/hat in school if significant photophobia: seat student away from bright windows and bright lights [] Reduce brightness on monitors/screens [] Change classroom seating to front of room as necessary
Auditory stimulus	[] Avoid loud classroom activities [] Lunch in a quiet place with a friend [] Avoid loud classes/places (music, band, choir, shop class, gym, cafeteria) [] Allow student to wear earplugs as needed [] Allow class transitions before the bell
School work	[] Simplify tasks (i.e., three-step instructions) [] Short breaks (5 min) between tasks [] Reduce overall amount of in class work [] Prorate workload (only core or important tasks) [] Reduce overall amount of in class work [] No homework [] Reduce amount of nightly homework [] Will attempt homework but will stop if symptoms occur [] Extra tutoring/assistance requested [] May begin make up of essential work
Testing	[] No testing [] Additional time for testing/untimed testing [] Alternative testing methods: oral delivery of questions, oral response, or scribe [] No more than one test per day [] No standardized testing
Education plan	[] Student is in need of a 504 plan and/or IEP (if prolonged symptoms are interfering with academic performance)

Question: How do you implement return to work?

The return-to-work (RTW) process, outlined in Table 10.4, is very similar to the return-to-learn protocol just discussed. Since work demands will vary significantly, an individualized approach is even more important in the work environment. After 24–48 h of relative brain rest including light mental activity, the patient may progress to part-time work, full-time work, and eventually full-time work with a normal workload. At each step the patient should progress if sustained mental activity does not worsen symptoms. Although the formal school supports seen in the return-to-learn protocol generally do not exist in the work environment, patients should have extra breaks, modified/ simplified tasks, extra time, and extended deadlines as they

Table 10.4 Return-to-work table [3, 4]

Phase	Activity	When to progress
1	Relative rest. Light mental exertion or work projects as tolerated. Limit screen time in first 48 h. Maximize sleep	24–48 h
2	Light mental activity. Up to 30 min of mental activity that does not worsen symptoms	Progress if 30 min of mental activity does not worsen symptoms
3	Part-time work with adjustments; breaks as needed, no formal presentations, modify/simplify tasks as needed, provide extra time for projects and modify deadlines if needed	Progress if 45 min of sustained mental activity does not worsen symptoms
4	Continue part-time work with moderate adjustments and begin to scale back extra time for projects as needed	Progress if 60 min of mental activity does not worsen symptoms
5	Attempt full-time work and continue to scale back occupation-specific accommodations	Progress if 60 min of mental activity does not cause symptoms and when accommodations are no longer needed
6	Full-time work with normal workload and no modifications	n/a

progress through the return-to-work process. Like students, workers may need light, noise and screen limitations, and restrictions depending on their symptom profile. If work tasks include manual labor or operating machinery, it is critical for the clinician to specify any physical activity limitations (such as limited driving, bending, or lifting heavy items while suffering from post-concussive dizziness). Clinicians may also use the return-to-play algorithm and testing of exercise tolerance to inform their recommendations. It is important to note, however, that these recommendations can be challenging for an employer to implement. Return to work may be nonlinear depending on these implementation challenges.

Question: When do you start progressing through the return to play and why is it necessary?

While return-to-learn and return-to-sport (RTS)strategies can run in parallel, a successful return to learn is necessary prior to completing the return-to-sport program [3]. Early data suggested that there is no standard physiological time window for SRC recovery, and research indicates that physiological dysfunction may outlast current clinical measures of recovery [23, 24]. Current research suggests this window could be better defined using universal definitions of recovery as described earlier in this chapter. The consequences of an athlete returning to sport with continued underlying physiologic dysfunction have yet to be understood fully, but possible outcomes of athletes returning to play while there is continued brain dysfunction include repeat injury, prolonged symptoms, increased risk of musculoskeletal injury, more severe physiologic dysfunction, or increased risk of neurodegenerative disease [25]. What is clearly understood is that initial symptom burden at time of first assessment (number and severity of symptoms) is the most predictive of longer

RTL and RTS. Likewise, continuing to play after concussion and delayed access to care are associated with prolonged recovery [3]. As such, a properly implemented return-to-play program serves as a buffer zone of gradually increasing activity before full-contact exposure risk.

The standard road to recovery after sports-related concussion follows a graduated stepwise rehabilitation strategy (an example is outlined in Table 10.5). The strategy starts with a 24–48 h period of initial relative rest that includes light activities of daily living, walking, and bursts of cognitive load while staying below the cognitive and physical threshold for exacerbating symptoms [3]. We explain to our patients and caregivers that symptoms are going to be present during the recovery period.

Once the patient is tolerating regular daily activities at school and home, we recommend starting supervised light aerobic activity (stage 2A) with the goal of increasing heart rate via walking or stationary cycling at a low to medium pace. This step is best coordinated with the athlete's certified athletic trainer (if available). Activities should be kept subthreshold, and any activity exacerbating symptoms should be discontinued. Athletes can progress up to stage 2B while completing the

Table 10.5 Example of return-to-play table [3, 4]

Stage	Aim	Activity	Goal of step
1	Symptom-limited activity	Daily activities that do not worsen symptoms including walking and brief cognitive loads starting 24–48 h after injury. Limit screen time in first 48 h. Maximize sleep	Gradual reintroduction of work and or school activities
2	Light aerobic exercise (2A)	Started after 24–48 h post SRC. Walking or stationary cycling at slow-to-medium pace; no resistance training	Keep HR below 55% of max predicted HR
	Moderate aerobic exercise (2B)	Walking, swimming, or stationary cycling at increased pace; light resistance training with bodyweight squats and pushups (one set of ten reps each)	Increase heart rate to 70% of maxHR
Return-to-learn protocol must be completed prior to advancing to stage 3			
3	Sports-specific exercise	Running and sports-specific drills away from team environment and activities without risk of head impact	Add movement and change of direction that challenges sensory motor systems
Medical determination of readiness to return to at-risk activities here			
4	Noncontact training drills	Harder drills (i.e., passing drills and return-to-team drills); may begin progressive resistance training and high-intensity exercise	Exercise, coordination, and increased thinking during sport
5	Full-contact practice	Participate in full/normal training activities	Restore confidence and allow coaching staff to assess functional skills
6	Return to sport	Normal unrestricted game play	Full clearance/participation

return-to-learn strategy. Once stage 2B is achieved, the athlete's symptoms have improved to a minimally symptomatic state, and they have completed a return-to-learn/return-to-work strategy and can progress to stage 3. If the athlete succeeds in navigating conditioning and sports-specific exercises defined for step 3, a medical determination of risk should be held. This risk assessment step should be completed prior to engaging in stage 4. A medical determination of risk discussion assesses the athlete's readiness for sports-related activities that have a higher risk of repeat concussion or exacerbating previous concussion symptoms due to their higher physical intensity and cognitive demands. An ideal candidate for continuing to stage 4 has completed RTL/RTW strategy, successfully navigated stages 1–3, and is adjudged to be clinically asymptomatic in their medical determination of risk. Athletes can then continue through the remaining stages of return to play until ready to be cleared for participation by their treating physician.

Each step of the return-to-play pathway should take at least 24 h to complete. This means that at least 1 week is required to progress through all stages of the protocol. "Thursday night clearance" is therefore not recommended, so high school football players who have a concussion on Friday night are not eligible to return to play the following Friday. The best athletes are at the highest risk of being returned too soon because coaches and parents often want them back out on the field early. Troy Aikman from the Dallas Cowboys specifically mentioned if he was the backup quarterback he would have had more time to rest from his frequent SRC. Because he was the starter, he felt he was encouraged and supported to return too quickly.

When implementing a return-to-play protocol, each patient's recovery is individual. We try to not place high expectations on a specific return to sport date, as this may cause increased stress and anxiety if actual recovery is not as fast as desired. It must be reiterated that the timeframe for the return-to-play protocol will vary based on an athlete's age, history, and level of sport. If the patient experiences any concussion-related symptoms during the stepwise return to play, then the athlete drops back to the previous asymptomatic level and attempts to progress again after being free of symptoms for another 24-h period at the lower level. If patients experience prolonged symptoms and resultant inactivity, each step may take longer than 24 h simply because of physical deconditioning that occurred during recovery. A great way to avoid this scenario is through a customized prescription for a symptom-limited exercise program. Of note if athletes experience new or worsening symptoms during recovery phase a new complete evaluation should be undertaken especcially if there are any red flags.

Historically, individualized sports-specific return-to-play protocols for sports with higher risk of head injury were developed to include a moderate activity phase highlighted by resistance training and contact drills specific to the athlete's sport. As of the 2022 CISG consensus statement however, this historical guidance was generalized to all sports by splitting step 2 into distinct phases, and instead adding a check point for discussion on when it is safe to advance to step 4 (noncontact sports-specific drills) and return to unrestricted sport (step 6) [4].

Question: How do you generate an exercise prescription? What is a Buffalo Concussion Treadmill test, and how is it useful?

To create an individualized exercise prescription, clinicians must be familiar with the Buffalo Concussion Treadmill Test (BCTT). The BCTT is a validated treadmill test that may be utilized to diagnose physiologic dysfunction in concussion patients [9, 26, 27]. As previously mentioned, it may be used to generate an individualized exercise prescription for those same patients suffering from prolonged concussion symptoms.

The BCTT may help differentiate concussion from other diagnoses such as cervical injury, vestibular/ocular dysfunction, depression, or posttraumatic headache syndrome such as migraines. If patients can exercise to exhaustion without reproduction or exacerbation of headache or other symptoms and they demonstrate a normal physiologic response to exercise, then symptoms are not likely due to sports-related concussion. It is also useful in quantifying the clinical severity and exercise capacity of concussed patients.

The test is based off the standard Balke cardiac treadmill test, which has been shown to be safe in patients with cardiac and orthopedic issues. A description of the Buffalo Treadmill Test can be found in Table 10.6. Absolute and relative contraindications are in Table 10.7. The starting speed is 3.6mph at 0% incline, but the starting speed can be slightly increased for taller or athletic persons and reduced for shorter or sedentary persons. During the first minute, the patient walks at 0% incline. The incline is increased to 1% at minute 2 and subsequently increased by 1% each minute thereafter. The speed remains constant until the maximum incline is reached or the patient cannot continue. Ratings of perceived exertion (using a Borg scale) and symptom score are assessed every minute (Fig. 10.1). Heart rate (by monitor) and blood pressure (by automated cuff) are measured every 2 min. The test is stopped with significant exacerbation of symptoms (defined as a 3-point increase from that

Table 10.6 Summary of buffalo treadmill test [26]

Test duration (minutes)	Speed (mph)	Incline (%)
First minute	3.6	0%
Second minute	3.6	1%
Subsequent minutes ➔ variation in incline		Incline is increased by 1% each minute until maximum incline is reached or stopping criteria fulfilled
Subsequent minutes ➔ variation in speed	If maximum incline is reached, then speed is increased by 0.4mph every minute until stopping criteria fulfilled	

Stopping criteria
1. Significant exacerbation of symptoms
    3-point increase from that day's pre-treadmill resting symptom sore on visual analog scale
2. Exhaustion
    RPE of 19–20 on Borg scale

Table 10.7 Absolute and relative contraindications to performing the BCTT [26]

Absolute contraindications to performing the BCTT	
History	Unwilling to exercise
	Increased risk for cardiopulmonary disease as defined by the ACSM[a]
Physical exam	Focal neurological deficit
	Significant balance deficit, visual deficit, or orthopedic injury that would represent a significant risk for walking/running on a treadmill
Relative contraindications to performing the BCTT	
History	Beta-blocker use
	Active major depression (may not comply with directions or prescription)
Physical exam	Minor balance deficit, visual deficit, or orthopedic injury that increases risk for walking/running on a treadmill (potential use of cycle ergometry)
	SBP >140mm Hg or DBP >90mm Hg
	Severe obesity

[a]Patients with known cardiovascular, pulmonary, or metabolic disease, signs and symptoms suggestive of cardiovascular or pulmonary disease, or individual aged >/= 45 years who have more than one risk factor to include: (1) family history of myocardial infarction, coronary revascularization, or sudden death before 55yr of age, (2) cigarette smoking, (3) hypertension, (4) hypercholesterolemia, (5) impaired fasting glucose, or (6) obesity

Rate Your Overall Condition

0	1-2	3-4	5-6	7-8	9-10
Feel terrific, no symptoms	Feel some symptoms but quite tolerable	Symptoms a little worse	Symptoms much worse	Feeling quite symptomatic	Feel terrible, worst I ever felt

Fig. 10.1 Visual analog symptom score scale [26]

day's pre-treadmill, resting, overall symptom score on a 1–10 point visual analog scale) or at exhaustion (RPE of 19–20 on the Borg scale). If the patient achieves the maximum incline without reaching either stopping criteria, then the treadmill speed is increased by 0.4mph every minute until stopping criteria are fulfilled. The test is deferred with any patient who has significant pretest resting symptoms defined as greater than or equal to 7 on the pretest visual analog scale. A sample visual analog scale can be seen in Fig. 10.1.

The BCTT may be used clinically to gauge recovery. If the patient can exercise to exhaustion (measured as reaching 85–90% of theoretic maximum HR) without symptom recurrence for 20 min, then it is safe to declare them physiologically recovered, and they can begin the graduated return-to-play protocol. Alternatively, if the patient develops symptoms prior to peak exertion, then you have objective evidence that the athlete is not physiologically ready and will need more recovery time. Per Leddy and Willer 2013, the most reported symptoms indicating that concussion has not resolved include worsening headache, dizziness/lightheaded-ness, and/or a sensation that the head feels full [26].

Additionally, the BCTT may be used to generate an exercise prescription while recovering. If a submaximal symptom exacerbation threshold is identified, then the patient is given a prescription to perform aerobic exercise on a stationary bicycle, treadmill, or elliptical for 20 min a day at subthreshold intensity (i.e., 80% of the threshold HR achieved on the BCTT) for 5–6 days per week. The BCTT may be repeated every 2–3 weeks to establish a new symptom-limited threshold HR. Alternatively, to avoid repeating the BCTT, once the practitioner has a baseline threshold HR and the patient is responding favorably, it is reasonable to increase the exercise HR target by 5–10 bpm every 2 weeks via phone or email. The BCTT is, however, not without risks or limitations. Concussed persons with orthopedic injuries like lower extremity fractures or those with baseline or concussive balance problems may not be able to safely complete the test [28]. Adaptive or para-athletes unable to stand may also find it difficult to complete the BCTT. Financial and staff limitations may also hamper the use of a BCTT, as not all clinics may have access to a treadmill on site or have additional trained staff such as physical therapists, athletic trainers, or other physicians to administer the test.

Depending on the individual needs of the concussed person or practical limitations discussed above, a buffalo bike test or standardized aerobic exercise (SAE) program can be implemented. The Buffalo Concussion Bike Test (BCBT) was developed by the same team as the BCTT to overcome some of the aforementioned limitations as well as expand opportunities for further research [28]. The BCBT follows the same progression as the BCTT described above with the following key differences (summarized in Table 10.8). Due to the longer time needed to reach a physiologic steady state heart rate on a stationary bike ergometer compared to a treadmill, the BCBT stages are 2 min in length as opposed to 1 min. Due to the change in load affecting the lower limb on a bike compared to a treadmill, the absolute workload for each bike stage was approximately 10% lower than the treadmill. By decreasing the load per stage, the BCBT prevented earlier fatigue/failure of the test on a bike than what would be expected on a treadmill. Most importantly, however, HR threshold on a bike and treadmill were found to be statistically equivalent at each level with the above adaptations [28]. To start the BCTB, participants begin cycling at 60 RPM with a set resistance based on their body mass. Resistance was then increased every 2 min until exhaustion or symptom exacerbation, following the same stop criteria as the BCTT.

Table 10.8 BCBT key differences		Activity
	1	2 min per stage rather than 1 min in BCTT
	2	10% less load per stage compared to BCTT

The Standardized Aerobic Exercise (SAE) program can be completed by an athlete and their entourage at home and without the need for treadmills or bike ergometers [29]. The SAE also affords athletes the freedom to choose their aerobic exercise so long as it does not pose a risk to their safety, is compatible with their symptoms profile, and the heart rate targets are reached [29]. To begin the program, athletes are assigned a target HR based on their sex assigned at birth and number of weeks since injury. Table 10.9 shows target HR as defined by the study which is approximately 90% of the expected HRt for that week and sex. Concussed persons are to exercise approximately 20 mins per day for 5–6 times per week at that target HR. If they can tolerate this, they may progress to the next level. If patients feel symptoms that are 2 or more points higher than their baseline, they should stop the activity and rest until the following day. This method has only been studied in adolescent athletes, however, and may have limited utility in other populations. Age does not seem to be a statistically significant factor in the adolescent age group.

Question: Why is return to play important to primary care providers and their patients?

Many concussions will only present to primary care providers and not providers well versed in concussion care. Regrettably, concussion management and recommendations continue to elude translation into practice. Recent surveys of both US and Canadian physicians continue to indicate that physical rest is the most commonly prescribed (erroneous) treatment for concussion [30, 31]. Cognitive rest and return-to-learn/return-to-play guidelines are also overlooked all together [30, 31].

How does return to learn and play look like for para-athletes?

Para-athletes encompass a large and diverse subset of athletes from recreational to elite levels who require an equally adaptive diagnosis and return-to-play/return-to-learn strategy. As a clinician caring for a para-athlete, a strong sense of their baseline must be identified. Some athletes may already experience headaches or balance perturbations as the norm. Others may not be able to see, hear, verbalize symptoms, or safely move their body as requiring a change in standard testing protocols. Wheelchair athletes, for instance, may need to change existing balance tests.

Table 10.9 HR prescriptions for standardized aerobic exercise for concussion recovery [29]

	Mean HR prescription
Females	
Week 1	116–119
Week 2	124–127
Week 3	132–135
Week 4	141–144
Males	
Week 1	123–126
Week 2	131–134
Week 3	140–143
Week 4	147–150

As described at the 2024 AMSSM national meeting, a wheelchair athlete may test their balance by holding a wheelie with eyes opened and closed. The first position statement for concussion in parasport offers more examples in their appendices [32]. As of this writing, studies have not validated the use of SCAT screening tools for any sub-type of para-athlete. Existing recommendations still encourage the use of current concussion guidelines as described above to the extent possible [32]. By establishing clear baseline symptom scores and creative concussion testing protocols, a para-athlete and their medical entourage can share in the decision-making regarding return to learn and play.

Key Points (Answers to Questions)
- Complete physical and mental rest is not recommended.
- Light activity should begin in the first 24–48 h.
- Individualized sub-symptom threshold aerobic exercise treatment may speed up recovery and reduce delayed recovery.
- Return-to-learn strategies include: (1) academic supports for transitioning back into the classroom and (2) formal interventions such as an individualized education plan (IEP) or a 504 plan if necessary.
- Return-to-learn/return-to-work and return-to-sport progressions can be implemented in parallel.
- Return-to-work progressions are tailored to symptom profiles and corresponding work specific tasks to ensure safe transitions.
- Buffalo Concussion Treadmill and Bike Tests can: (1) generate individualized exercise prescriptions, (2) assess physiologic recovery, and (3). help differentiate concussion from other diagnoses.
- Return to sports specific activity with a team is done after a medical evaluation of risk.
- A minimum of 1 week/24 h between stages is needed (no Thursday night clearance).
  Unrestricted return to sport is attempted when: (1) no concussion-related symptoms from the current concussion are present, (2) after return-to-learn/ return-to-work pathway, and (3) after return-to-sport pathway.
- Para-athletes may require adaptations to concussion testing/rehabilitation given degree of ability and baseline symptoms.

References

1. Thomas D, Apps J, Hoffmann R, McCrea M, Hammeke T. Benefits of strict rest after acute concussion: a randomized controlled trial. Pediatrics. 2015;135:213–23.
2. Grool A, Aglipay M, Momoli F, Meehan W, Freedman S, Yeates K, et al. Association between early participation in physical activity following acute concussion and persistent postconcussive symptoms in children and adolescents. JAMA. 2016;316(23):2504.
3. Putukian M, Purcell L, Schneider KJ, et al. Clinical recovery from concussion–return to school and sport: a systematic review and meta-analysis. Br J Sports Med. 2023;57:798–809.

4. Patricios JS, Schneider KJ, Dvorak J, et al. Consensus statement on concussion in sport: the 6th International Conference on Concussion in Sport–Amsterdam, October 2022. Br J Sports Med. 2023;57:695–711.
5. Craton N, Leslie O. Is rest the best intervention for concussion? Lessons learned from the whiplash model. Curr Sports Med Rep. 2014;13:201–4.
6. McCauley S, Boake C, Levin H, Contant C, Song J. Postconcussional disorder following mild to moderate traumatic brain injury: anxiety, depression, and social support as risk factors and comorbidities. J Clin Exp Neuropsychol. 2001;23:792–808.
7. Halstead M, Eagan Brown B, McAvoy K. Cognitive rest following concussions: rethinking 'cognitive rest'. Br J Sports Med. 2016;51(3):147.
8. Brooks B, Low T, Daya H, Khan S, Mikrogianakis A, Barlow K. Test or Rest? Computerized Cognitive Testing in the Emergency Department after Pediatric Mild Traumatic Brain Injury Does Not Delay Symptom Recovery. J Neurotrauma. 2016;33:2091–6.
9. Leddy J, Hinds A, Miecznikowski J, Darling S, Matuszak J, Baker J, et al. Safety and prognostic utility of provocative exercise testing in acutely concussed adolescents. Clin J Sport Med. 2018;28(1):13–20.
10. Leddy J, Haider M, Ellis M, Mannix R, Darling S, Freitas M, et al. Early subthreshold aerobic exercise for sport-related concussion. JAMA Pediatr. 2019;
11. Alla S, Sullivan S, McCrory P. Defining asymptomatic status following sports concussion: fact or fallacy? Br J Sports Med. 2011;46:562–9.
12. Haider M, Leddy J, Pavlesen S, Kluczynski M, Baker J, Miecznikowski J, et al. A systematic review of criteria used to define recovery from sport-related concussion in youth athletes. Br J Sports Med. 2017;52(18):1179–90.
13. Covassin T, Elbin R, Harris W, Parker T, Kontos A. The role of age and sex in symptoms, neurocognitive performance, and postural stability in athletes after concussion. Am J Sports Med. 2012;40(6):1303–12.
14. Yeates KO, Räisänen AM, Premji Z, et al. What tests and measures accurately diagnose persisting post-concussive symptoms in children, adolescents and adults following sport-related concussion? A systematic review. Br J Sports Med. 2023;57:780–8.
15. Schneider KJ, Critchley ML, Anderson V, Davis GA, Debert CT, Feddermann-Demont N, Gagnon I, Guskiewicz KM, Hayden KA, Herring S, Johnstone C, Makdissi M, Master CL, Moser RS, Patricios JS, Register-Mihalik JK, Ronksley PE, Silverberg ND, Yeates KO. Targeted interventions and their effect on recovery in children, adolescents and adults who have sustained a sport-related concussion: a systematic review. Br J Sports Med. 2023;57(12):771–9. https://doi.org/10.1136/bjsports-2022-106685.
16. Leddy JJ, Burma JS, Toomey CM, Hayden A, Davis GA, Babl FE, Gagnon I, Giza CC, Kurowski BG, Silverberg ND, Willer B, Ronksley PE, Schneider KJ. Rest and exercise early after sport-related concussion: a systematic review and meta-analysis. Br J Sports Med. 2023;57(12):762–70. https://doi.org/10.1136/bjsports-2022-106676.
17. Meehan WP 3rd, d'Hemecourt P, Collins CL, Taylor AM, Comstock RD. Computerized neurocognitive testing for the management of sport-related concussions. Pediatrics. 2012;129:38–44.
18. Van Kampen D, Lovell M, Pardini J, Collins M, Fu H. The "value added" of neurocognitive testing after sports-related concussion. Am J Sports Med. 2006;34:1630–5.
19. Harmon K, Clugston J, Dec K, Hainline B, Herring S, Kane S, et al. American medical society for sports medicine position statement on concussion in sport. Clin J Sport Med. 2019;29(2):87–100.
20. Wasserman E, Bazarian J, Mapstone M, Block R, van Wijngaarden E. Academic dysfunction after a concussion among US high school and college students. Am J Public Health. 2016;106(7):1247–53.
21. Russell K, Hutchison M, Selci E, Leiter J, Chateau D, Ellis M. Academic outcomes in high-school students after a concussion: a retrospective population-based analysis. PLoS One. 2016;11(10):e0165116.

22. McAvoy K, Eagan-Johnson B, Halstead M. Return to learn: transitioning to school and through ascending levels of academic support for students following a concussion. Neuro Rehabil. 2018;42(3):325–30.
23. Prichep L, McCrea M, Barr W, Powell M, Chabot R. Time course of clinical and electrophysiological recovery after sport-related concussion. J Head Trauma Rehabil. 2013;28:266–73.
24. Wang Y, Nelson L, LaRoche A, Pfaller A, Nencka A, Koch K, et al. Cerebral blood flow alterations in acute sport-related concussion. J Neurotrauma. 2016;33:1227–36.
25. Kamins J, Bigler E, Covassin T, Henry L, Kemp S, Leddy J, et al. What is the physiological time to recovery after concussion? A systematic review. Br J Sports Med. 2017;51:935–40.
26. Leddy J, Willer B. Use of graded exercise testing in concussion and return-to-activity management. Curr Sports Med Rep. 2013;12(6):370–6.
27. Cordingley D, Girardin R, Reimer K, Ritchie L, Leiter J, Russell K, et al. Graded aerobic treadmill testing in pediatric sports-related concussion: safety, clinical use, and patient outcomes. J Neurosurg Pediatr. 2016;18(6):693–702.
28. Haider MN, Johnson SL, Mannix R, Macfarlane AJ, Constantino D, Johnson BD, Willer B, Leddy J. The buffalo concussion bike test for concussion assessment in adolescents. Sports Health. 2019;11(6):492–7. https://doi.org/10.1177/1941738119870189.
29. Chizuk HM, Haider MN, Edmonds JQ, Rawlings A, Willer BS, Leddy JJ. Practical management: a standardized aerobic exercise program for adolescents with concussion in the absence of graded exercise testing. Clin J Sport Med. 2023;33(3):276–9. https://doi.org/10.1097/JSM.0000000000001116.
30. Lebrun C, Mrazik M, Prasad A, Tjarks B, Dorman J, Bergeron M, et al. Sport concussion knowledge base, clinical practices and needs for continuing medical education: a survey of family physicians and cross-border comparison. Br J Sports Med. 2012;47(1):54–9.
31. Zemek R, Eady K, Moreau K, Farion K, Solomon B, Weiser M, et al. Canadian pediatric emergency physician knowledge of concussion diagnosis and initial management. CJEM. 2015;17(02):115–22.
32. Weiler R, Blauwet C, Clarke D, et al. Concussion in para sport: the first position statement of the Concussion in Para Sport (CIPS) Group. Br J Sports Med. 2021;55:1187–95.

Chapter 11
Post-concussion Syndrome: Persistent Post-concussive Symptoms (PPCS) or Persistent Symptoms after Concussion (PSaC)

Landan Banks, Nathan Howell, and Jack Spittler

Clinical Case

A 17-year-old high school athlete missed the majority of the fall soccer season due to a concussion she sustained in the second game. She is considering trying out for track and field but still suffers from headaches 4 months later and simply does not feel as competitive as she used to. She wants to know if these symptoms are due to her concussion and what she can do to feel better before the spring tryouts.

When does a concussion evolve into post-concussion syndrome?

There is no consensus definition for post-concussion syndrome—making diagnosis, treatment, and broader scientific study a challenge. Historically, the most commonly used diagnostic criteria come from the *Diagnostic and Statistical Manual of Mental Disorders* (DSM-4) and the *International Statistical Classification of Diseases and Related Health Problems* (ICD-10). The updated DSM-5 has abandoned its former classification system and now the greater scientific community has adopted the more clinically relevant term "persistent post-concussive symptoms" (PPCS) [1, 2].

DSM Criteria

Previously, the DSM-4 utilized the term "post-concussional disorder." In short, this diagnosis required that cognitive impairment plus a certain amount of new or worsening specific symptoms occurs after a concussion, causing some degree of

L. Banks · N. Howell · J. Spittler (✉)
University of Colorado School of Medicine, Denver, CO, USA
e-mail: john.spittler@cuanschutz.edu

© The Author(s), under exclusive license to Springer Nature
Switzerland AG 2025
D. S. Patel (ed.), *Concussion Management for Primary Care*,
https://doi.org/10.1007/978-3-031-85516-0_11

disability for at least 3 months [1]. The DSM-5 discards this term in favor of "major or mild neurocognitive disorder due to traumatic brain injury." Under these criteria, there must be evidence of a traumatic brain injury with at least one of the following: loss of consciousness, posttraumatic amnesia, disorientation and confusion, or other neurologic signs. In the immediate period following the injury, the patient must also demonstrate a decline in at least one of six cognitive domains: complex attention, executive function, learning and memory, language, perceptual motor, or social cognition. This disorder is designated as either mild or major based on the severity of symptoms and degree of functional deficit. Although specific symptom durations are not required for diagnosis, the DSM-5 suggests that symptoms lasting beyond 3 months exceeds the expected recovery time of a concussion [3].

ICD-10 Criteria

The ICD-10 uses the terminology "post-concussional syndrome." Postconcussional syndrome is defined as a history of traumatic brain injury (TBI) that is usually severe enough to cause loss of consciousness and is followed by three or more of the following eight features: headache, dizziness, fatigue, irritability, insomnia, difficulty concentrating, memory deficits, and decreased tolerance to stress, emotion, or alcohol [2].

Persistent Post-concussive Symptoms (PPCS)

The prior criteria have varying requirements for symptom duration, initial injury, symptomatology, and objective findings. These discrepancies make it difficult to determine which patients warrant further evaluation and when this evaluation should occur. As a result, the 5th and 6th International Conference on Concussion in Sport and the American Medical Society for Sports Medicine favor the term persistent post-concussive symptoms (PPCS), which is the term that will be utilized for the remainder of this chapter [4–6]. Patients with PPCS experience symptoms that extend beyond the expected recovery time of 2 weeks for adults and 4 weeks for children. This patient-centric diagnosis captures all patients who do not recover as anticipated following a concussion—targeting this population for further evaluation and treatment.

Who is at risk for developing post-concussion symptoms?

The majority of adults and older adolescents (~80–90%) will achieve clinical recovery from a concussion within 2 weeks, while the majority of children and younger adolescents may require up to 4 weeks to return to baseline [7, 8]. The remaining ~10–15% of patients will experience PPCS ranging from weeks to years following their initial injury [9]. Identifying patients at risk for developing PPCS is important so that aggressive and individualized treatment strategies can be employed to reduce the duration of symptoms and burden of disability. A great deal of effort has been dedicated to identifying such risk factors; however, many results have been inconsistent. Heterogeneous diagnostic criteria (as described above) make it difficult to compare and pool research. Overall, however, it appears that increased initial symptom burden and severity, female sex, adolescent age, preinjury mental health diagnoses and specific post-injury symptoms such as headache, migraine, dizziness, oculomotor dysfunction, and depression may all increase the risk of prolonged recovery [8, 10, 11]. Of note, patients with learning disabilities or attention-deficit/hyperactivity disorder are not known to be at greater risk for developing PPCS [10].

What causes persistent symptoms following a concussion?

Knowledge of acute concussion pathophysiology continues to grow. It is thought that temporary mechanical forces on neurons incite a cascade of events that include inappropriate ion shifts, diffuse neuronal depolarization, abnormal neurotransmitter release, autoregulatory disturbances and altered cerebral blood flow (CBF), neuro-inflammation, and metabolic mismatch and depression. It is postulated that axonal injury, impaired neuroplasticity, blood-brain barrier dysfunction, and even some degree of cell death may also play a role in concussion [12]. Alternatively, the exact pathophysiology of PPCS remains unknown. It has been hypothesized that continued physiologic derangements, neuro-inflammation, axonal injury, whiplash injury, vestibulo-ocular dysfunction, and psychological factors may all be contributors [13].

Physiologic Derangements

Persistent physiologic derangements such as autonomic, CBF, and metabolic dysfunction have been postulated as causes of PPCS. This idea is extrapolated from the better-known pathophysiology of acute concussion and based on the observation that some patients with PPCS experience symptoms largely with physical or cognitive exertion rather than at rest [14]. Indeed, higher resting heart rates following TBI and increased heart rates during cognitive exertion in PPCS suggest continued autonomic dysfunction in this patient population [15, 16]. The role of CBF dysfunction is less certain. Reduced CBF is found in 40–60% of patients with PPCS using single positron emission computed tomography (SPECT) [9]. Interestingly, similar findings have been noted in disease states such as neck and back pain, whiplash injuries, obsessive-compulsive disorder, depression, chronic fatigue, AIDS dementia complex, and more [17–23]. In light of its seeming ubiquity in other disorders, it is uncertain whether CBF dysfunction plays a causative role in PPCS. Similarly, available evidence does not clearly support metabolic dysfunction as a cause of PPCS. Research utilizing magnetic resonance spectroscopy demonstrates reduced N-acetyl aspartate (NAA) (a correlate of ATP) in patients with PPCS; however, these metabolic changes are also seen in asymptomatic patients who have recovered

appropriately from a concussion—calling to question the strength of the relationship between symptomology and metabolic dysfunction in PPCS as measured by
NAA [9, 24, 25]. This does not disprove that continued metabolic depression has a
role in PPCS but may rather demonstrate that a more indicative biomarker has not
been found.

Neuro-inflammation

Neuro-inflammation may also contribute to PPCS. Increased levels of the serum
inflammatory marker, C-reactive protein (CRP), are associated with PPCS as well
as persistent cognitive dysfunction and psychological issues following TBI [26]. It
has also been considered that systemic inflammation—even in the absence of TBI—
may be the true underlying source of PPCS-like symptoms. In this model, concussion is merely one of many possible inciting etiologies [27]. This concept is in part
based upon research showing that post-concussive symptoms occur after both concussion and poly-trauma without brain injury [28]. It must be noted, however, that
this study evaluated symptoms within 2 weeks of initial injuries and therefore,
results may not be generalizable to timeframes typically encompassed by PPCS
(>2–4 weeks). More specific markers of inflammation have been evaluated, including interleukin-8, interleukin-9, and platelet-derived growth factor at various times
after injury. They may hold some prognostic value; however, availability of these
studies could limit wide application [29]. Overall, more research is needed to elucidate the relationship between inflammation and PPCS. Better understanding of this
potential pathophysiology may lead to integration of biomarkers into clinical prediction models and novel anti-inflammatory treatments for PPCS in the future.

Axonal Injury

It has also been theorized that axonal dysfunction contributes to PPCS. In acute
concussion, rapid head deceleration produces shearing forces that can result in
structural axonal damage, subsequently increased calcium, and resultant axonal
dysfunction [9]. Diffusion tensor imaging (DTI) shows that patients who suffer a
concussion demonstrate white matter changes beyond expected recovery times
compared to patients with non-brain injuries (cervical injuries excluded). This is
being investigated as a potential tool to help with early prediction of patients at risk
for prolonged recovery [30]. Interestingly, these concussion-related white matter
changes are present in patients who develop PPCS as well as those who do not [31].
These results suggest that continued axonal dysfunction does not appear to play a
role in PPCS.

Whiplash Injury

It is likely that whiplash injuries often occur concurrently with concussions and therefore may play a role in PPCS. Isolated whiplash injuries and concussions share many associated symptoms such as headache, neck pain, nausea/vomiting, dizziness, instability, vision changes, memory deficits, decreased concentration, and more [9]. Limited research shows that when compared to controls, patients with PPCS suffer higher levels of painful upper cervical joint dysfunction, reduced neck flexor endurance, and increased neck spasm [32]. Furthermore, patients with PPCS experience significant pain relief from therapies directed at the cervical spine such as cervical mobilization and assisted muscle-stretching therapy [33]. Cervicovestibular rehabilitation therapy for persistent post-concussive symptoms such as neck pain, headache, and/or dizziness results in a dramatic increase in patients who are able to return to sport [34]. Whiplash may further contribute to persistent post-concussive symptoms by altering cervical proprioception. Cervical muscle and joint mechanoreceptors feed proprioceptive information to multiple levels of the central nervous system (CNS) and are responsible for informing the cervicocollic, vestibulocollic, and cervico-ocular reflexes. These reflexes work to stabilize the head during complex movements [14]. Although the mechanisms behind cervical proprioceptive dysfunction remain unknown, it is postulated that alterations therein could lead to common concussion symptoms such as dizziness and imbalance. Taken together, these results expose the possibility that some persistent post-concussive symptoms may have a cervicogenic etiology.

Vestibulo-ocular Dysfunction

Dysfunction of the vestibulo-ocular system (VOS) may also contribute to PPCS [14]. The VOS consists of peripheral inputs from the inner ears, eyes, and musculoskeletal mechanoreceptors that feed processing centers in the CNS [35]. Efferent signals from the CNS then complete pathways for important reflexes such as the vestibulo-ocular reflex (VOR) and the vestibulo-spinal reflex (VSR). The VOR coordinates fixed gaze during head acceleration. The VSR consists of compensatory body movements induced by changes in head position to maintain balance and posture. Like other potential causes of PPCS, the pathophysiology of persistent VOS dysfunction after concussion is not fully understood; however, complications such as labyrinthine concussion, perilymphatic fistula, endolymphatic hydrops, or central vestibular lesions may be contributors [36, 37]. It seems logical that alterations of this complex system could account for persistent post-concussive symptoms such as dizziness, imbalance, fogginess, nausea/vomiting, blurred vision, headache, and "not feeling right" [5].

Psychological Dysfunction

Finally, it is likely that psychological factors have an etiologic role in persistent post-concussive symptoms, as suggested by the increased risk of developing PPCS in those with underlying mental health diagnoses [38]. In some patients, persistent post-concussion symptoms may include depressed mood, anxiety, irritability, decreased concentration, fatigue, and sleep disturbances. In these situations, it may be difficult to determine whether symptoms are due to a concussion or from a pre-existing psychological disorder. This highlights the importance of knowing a patient's baseline mental health status and diagnoses. More research is needed to define relative risk for distinct mental health diagnoses and for severity of psychological symptoms and treatment status at the time of concussion [39].

How can a clinician evaluate persistent post-concussive symptoms?

It is important to understand that persistent post-concussion symptoms usually have several contributing etiologies—as described above—resulting in heterogeneous clinical presentations. "Clinical profiles" are a developing concept in concussion care that reflect this. These profiles categorize symptoms as cognitive/fatigue, oculomotor, vestibular, cervical, migraine, and anxiety/mood [14, 40, 41] (Table 11.1). Symptoms may be unique to one profile or shared. These profiles provide a conceptual framework for evaluation and treatment of PPCS.

As with acute concussion, evaluation starts with a thorough history of the initial injury and following events. Clinical inventories such as the symptom checklist on the Sports Concussion Assessment Tool Sixth Edition (SCAT6) can help identify and track the progression of collective post-concussive symptoms [42]. Designed to assist in the multimodal examination of athletes, this tool is most effective in discriminating between concussed and non-concussed athletes within 72 hours of injury and up to 7 days post-injury, although its clinical utility appears to diminish after 72 hours. The diminished sensitivity of this assessment tool may result from ceiling effects, low test-retest reliability, and/or other psychometric issues. Except for the post-concussion symptom scale (PCSS), these findings suggest that the

Table 11.1 Possible symptoms in PPCS

Musculoskeletal	Whiplash/cervical dysfunction
Psychologic	Anxiety Depression Concentration difficulties
Neurologic	Vestibulo-ocular dysfunction Dizziness Photophobia Phonophobia Headaches Memory problems
Other	Sleep disturbance Fatigue/exercise intolerance

SCAT tools may not be appropriate for use in the return-to-sport (RTS) decision-making process beyond 7 days post-injury [42]. It also does not prompt evaluation of all of the phenotypes of a concussion [43].

While there is an absence of an objective, gold-standard criterion for the diagnosis and evaluation of prolonged post-concussion syndrome, consensus does exist on effectiveness of an interdisciplinary, biopsychosocial approach based on individualized symptom profile [44]. Newer assessment tools, such as the Concussion Office Based Rehabilitation Assessment (COBRA), provide a comprehensive method of assessing the patient in the office, not in the milieu of sport. It is designed to identify most manifestations of concussion and further assessment of all potential concussion phenotypes [43].

A complete physical examination should be done with special attention to the neurologic and vestibulo-ocular systems, the cervical spine, and cognition. (See chapter on Concussion Physical Exam for further details.) Focal findings warrant advanced imaging; however, the neurologic exam will be unremarkable in the vast majority of patients with PPCS [45].

Clinical profiles, as mentioned above, may help guide further testing. Formal and computerized neuropsychological testing measure cognitive deficits [46]. The Beck Depression Inventory-II (BDI-II), Patient Health Questionnaire (PHQ-9), and Brief Symptom Inventory-18 (BSI-18) evaluate affective symptoms [46]. Exercise testing with the Buffalo concussion treadmill test and autonomic evaluation with tilt table testing can help detect physiologic dysfunction [46].

Structural imaging such as standard CT and MRI are generally uninformative in PPCS evaluation. Functional MRI, diffusion tensor imaging, magnetic resonance spectroscopy, and quantitative EEG have all demonstrated measurable differences in patients with PPCS versus controls. This is important in the research setting; however, results often do not change clinical management. Similarly, genetic testing and biomarkers continue to be subjects of study but do not yet have a role in clinical medicine [46].

Finally, it is important to remember that if a patient is not recovering as expected following a concussion, preexisting and alternative diagnoses—apart from PPCS—should also be considered.

What is the best approach to treatment of prolonged concussion symptoms?

Treatment for prolonged concussion symptoms has traditionally been based on an extension of the guidelines for treating acute concussion or those used in treating mild traumatic brain injury (TBI) [47]. This is usually not effective for prolonged symptoms, however, since treatment for acute concussion usually consists of a more general approach with a brief period of rest, followed by light exercise and gradual return to activity as symptoms improve. Current evidence suggests that management of prolonged symptoms should focus on active treatment of specific primary and secondary diagnoses identified on assessment. Recent systematic reviews have advocated use of somatic, cognitive, mental health, physiological (exercise), cervical spine, vestibular, oculomotor, autonomic, sleep, hormonal, and loss of cognitive and/or physical stamina in the assessment in order to facilitate individualized and targeted management of post-concussion syndrome [46] (Table 11.2). It is ideal for those with PPCS to be evaluated by a provider or multidisciplinary team with expertise in complicated concussion management [5]. A collaborative treatment approach that includes exercise, therapy, mental health, and possibly pharmacotherapy can be then utilized. Further high-quality studies are still needed, but there are some good data to help guide treatment for prolonged concussion symptoms.

Exercise

Initially the mainstay of treatment for concussion was "cocoon therapy" which involved complete rest with avoidance of activity and stimulation [48, 49]. Especially for prolonged concussion symptoms, there is emerging evidence that voluntary and controlled exercise, not rest, is a much better treatment option. Exercise intolerance may actually be a physiologic biomarker of an ongoing concussion and return of normal exercise tolerance may help to establish recovery from a concussion [50]. An individualized, symptom-limited aerobic exercise program has been shown to be safe and effective in improving persistent symptoms compared to controls [51–53]. One such program is the Buffalo Concussion Exercise Treatment Protocol. This is a progressive sub-symptom threshold aerobic exercise program based upon systematically establishing the level of exercise tolerance on the Buffalo Concussion Treadmill Test (BCCT), which is the most studied, controlled exercise program [54]. Along these lines, there is also evidence that inactivity may prolong concussion symptoms, such as vestibular dysfunction and depression/anxiety [55, 56].

Table 11.2 Potential referrals for PPCS

Referral	Reasons for referral
Neuropsychology or psychology	Neuropsychological evaluation
	Depression, anxiety, or other psych symptoms
Psychiatry	Depression, anxiety, or other psych symptoms
Neurology	Headaches
	Dizziness/vestibular dysfunction
	Memory issues
Ophthalmology	Oculomotor dysfunction
Optometry	Light/vision dysfunction
Sleep medicine	Sleep disturbance
Physical or occupational therapy	Cervical dysfunction
	Balance issues
	Impaired activities of daily living (ADLs)

Vestibular and Oculomotor/Vision Therapy

Vestibular and oculomotor symptoms occur in about 60% of athletes with sports-related post-concussive symptoms [57, 58]. This may include dizziness, vertigo, disequilibrium, impaired balance, blurry/unstable vision, and nausea. Presence of these symptoms at time of injury, especially dizziness, is predictive of a prolonged concussion recovery [59]. Therapy should focus on specific deficits identified and utilize an "expose-recover" model performed by clinicians with expertise in vestibular rehabilitation [60, 61]. There is some evidence that addressing vestibular dysfunction with a targeted physical therapy program improves outcomes in those with post-concussive symptoms [34, 62].

The control of eye movements is guided by several parts of the brain that are particularly vulnerable to concussion [63]. Physical examination may reveal deficits in saccades, anti-saccades, smooth visual pursuits, vergence, accommodation, vestibular-ocular reflex, visual fields, and photosensitivity. The most commonly diagnosed vision problems in athletes with PPCS are convergence insufficiency (CI) and accommodative insufficiency (AI) [64]. If there is a deficit, referral to an eye care specialist (optometrist or ophthalmologist) should be considered. Therapy directed at certain ocular deficits or more general oculomotor training (OMT) is shown to be beneficial for individuals with oculomotor issues with PPCS [65, 66]. Emerging evidence suggests that virtual reality is an effective tool for the rehabilitation of vestibular and balance impairments post-concussion. More research is necessary to develop a quantitative standard and to better understand appropriate dosage of virtual reality intervention [67].

Light Therapy

Light affects many aspects of human physiology including circadian rhythm, sleep-wake cycles, alertness, cognition, and mood. There is some evidence that light therapy may be helpful in treating PPCS. Athletes with concussion who receive daily blue-wavelength light therapy have shown decreased daytime fatigue, improved sleep, greater alertness, and reduced anxiety compared to controls [68–70]. In addition, emerging evidence suggests that green light may be an effective sleep promoter and reduce headache symptoms, while red light may aid in alertness [68, 71]. Mitigation of certain light wavelengths may also be helpful. In one small study of athletes with photophobia following concussion, 85% experienced symptom relief when using glasses of one or more colors. The colors that provided the most relief were blue, green, red, and purple, and no adverse events were reported [72]. Furthermore, in a small study from 2020, 35 adults with mild TBI (mTBI) were given 6-week morning blue-light therapy and compared with a control group. The blue-light therapy group showed significant improvement in sleep, daytime sleepiness, depression, PCS, and executive functions [73]. More investigation is needed in regards to light therapy for treatment of PPCS, as it may be an inexpensive, yet effective treatment with minimal side effects.

Physical/Occupational Therapy

As mentioned earlier, concomitant injury to the cervical spine (resembling whiplash) may occur with concussion [74]. The neck and upper cervical spine are particularly vulnerable to injury as they are the most mobile part of the vertebral column. Cervical spine injuries have been linked with headache, blurry vision, dizziness, and vertigo, and therefore these symptoms of a concussion may be derived from injury to the brain, neck, or both [75]. If neck pathology is felt to be contributing to PPCS, the athlete should be referred to physical therapy with focus on neck position, manual therapy, neuromotor/sensorimotor retraining, and postural stability [76].

Headaches

In many cases, it can be difficult to distinguish PPCS from a primary headache disorder. Athletes with prolonged headache following concussion should be evaluated for underlying headache disorders, cervical dysfunction causing headache, and other possible contributors [46]. Obtaining a thorough history of previous headache disorders and treatment is essential with special attention paid to any differences in symptomatology. Pharmacologic treatment of prolonged concussion-related headaches often mimics that of chronic migraines and may include prophylactic treatment with tricyclic anti-depressants (TCAs, i.e., nortriptyline), beta blockers (i.e., propranolol), and anticonvulsants (i.e., gabapentin) and/or abortive treatment with NSAIDs, acetaminophen, and triptans [77]. Both gabapentin and TCAs have immediate impact on symptom burden following concussion; however, they are not proven to reduce symptoms in PPCS [78]. Medications such as these may have side effects including dizziness, drowsiness, and blurry vision, which could potentially exacerbate other PPCS symptoms. Therefore, they should be used very judiciously and with close monitoring of symptoms. Athletes with PPCS should be asked about current medication use (including over-the-counter medications)—medication, dose, and frequency. The athlete may be overusing medications, which could exacerbate symptoms or cause rebound headaches. It has been shown that greater initial PPCS scores result in higher likelihood of receiving medications for treatment, which may not be helpful or even detrimental in PPCS treatment [79]. Non-pharmacological approaches to treatment of headaches secondary to PPCS have also been studied, including cognitive-behavioral therapy (CBT) and manual therapy with varying efficacy [73]. Studies focused on the effects of repetitive transcranial magnetic stimulation (rTMS) on headaches have shown mostly positive results thus far [73, 80].

Sleep Disturbance

High-quality sleep has emerged as an incredibly important factor in athletics and many other aspects of human performance. Sleep disruption is a common symptom in athletes with PPCS. Prevalence and severity are not well studied, but some data show that sleep disturbance may be present in over half of athletes with slow recovery from concussion [81]. Problems with sleep may be associated with higher overall symptom severity burden, balance disturbance (modified Balance Error Scoring System (mBESS)), and worsened reaction time during recovery [82, 83]. In addition, history of repeated concussion is associated with longer concussion duration and higher reported sleep disturbance. Those athletes with sleep disturbance also exhibit more severe headaches, mood disturbance, and cognitive dysfunction [84]. In athletes with sleep disturbance, sleep hygiene should first be addressed [85]. This may include enacting a regular daily bedtime, avoiding stimulating activities immediately before bed, not consuming caffeine for 4–6 hours prior to bedtime, and avoiding daytime naps, among other strategies. CBT and psychological support have been shown to improve sleep quality after mild traumatic brain injury (mTBI) [73, 86–88]. Light therapy may also be helpful [89, 90]. Pharmacotherapy should be used judiciously as most medication use is off-label to treat sleep following concussion. Medications may include analgesics, muscle relaxants, melatonin, and hypnotics. While not all of the reasons are clear, reduced evening melatonin production may be present in the body following concussion, which could consequently alter circadian rhythm [91]. There is, however, no conclusive evidence that melatonin is beneficial in sleep disturbance in PPCS [92]. While melatonin may be well-tolerated and improve sleep duration and quality, it does not reduce post-concussive symptom severity or duration [93–95]. Sedatives should be avoided but, if used, only for a short (2–3 week) period. Antidepressants may be considered to treat sleep, especially if concurrent mood alterations are present [96].

Psychological Symptoms

Individuals experiencing prolonged psychological symptoms such as irritability, sadness, and anxiety after a concussion should be evaluated further and offered appropriate treatment. These symptoms (especially if untreated) may lead to depression, post-traumatic stress disorder, and behavioral disorders, which can be short- and longer-term sequelae of concussion [85, 97, 98]. It has been shown that a collaborative care model can improve outcomes in those with prolonged psychological symptoms [99]. An important initial intervention can simply be discussing the concussion diagnosis and prognosis more thoroughly with the individual and their family or providing them with educational materials. Reassurance, discussing expected recovery time, and education about coping strategies have been shown to improve PPCS [100]. Non-pharmacologic treatment options also include cognitive-behavioral therapy (CBT). There is some limited evidence that CBT may help treat post-concussive symptoms and reduce or prevent PPCS in individuals who are "at-risk" (initial high symptom severity and belief that symptoms will persist) for developing PPCS [101, 102]. Neuropsychological evaluation should be considered early on in PPCS if psychological symptoms are present. Neuropsychologists can provide biopsychosocial evaluation and treatment services to nonathletes and athletes. In athletes, they are able to provide post-injury education and emotional reassurance, guidance on symptom management and emotional support, and assistance with return-to-play and return-to-school processes [103]. Safe exercise and rehabilitation programs (including low-intensity aerobic exercise, sports drills, relaxation exercises) may result in decreased anxiety and "anger" in athletes with PPCS [44].

Pharmacologic therapy can be directed at the type of psychological disturbance. Generally, selective serotonin reuptake inhibitors (SSRIs) are recommended as first-line treatment if depression and anxiety symptoms are present post-concussion. Efficacy and tolerability of serotonin and norepinephrine reuptake inhibitors (SNRIs) are less established, but expert consensus guidelines endorse their use for these symptoms. Tricyclic antidepressants (i.e., amitriptyline) may be considered, especially if there are concomitant headache issues, but should be used cautiously due to a less favorable risk-benefit profile [104]. A different pharmacologic therapy can be considered if the main psychological symptoms are related to attention difficulties. In a meta-analysis of randomized controlled trials, methylphenidate (stimulant used for ADHD/ADD treatment) was found to be effective for attention deficits after mTBI [105]. Comorbid fatigue, daytime sleepiness, and apathy may also respond favorably to stimulant treatment [106, 107]. As stimulants may have significant side effects (poor appetite, insomnia, weight loss, etc.) and could result in dependence, they should be used very judiciously with careful monitoring of symptoms.

What are the potential complications associated with prolonged post-concussion symptoms?

Second Impact Syndrome

Second impact syndrome is a controversial condition in which an individual experiences a second head injury prior to full recovery from the initial head injury. This is a rare, but catastrophic, complication that could result from returning an individual too quickly to athletics. If after a concussion the athlete is still symptomatic, this indicates that the brain is still in a fragile state due to altered cerebral metabolism. A second impact during this period could potentially cause complete dysregulation of cerebral perfusion and pressure control. This leads to rapid swelling in the brain and increased intracranial pressure, consequently leading to brain herniation and death. It is likely that triggering the trigemino-cardiac reflex is a crucial element in explaining the sequence of clinical events and its association with a state of neurogenic inflammation [108]. Because it is so rare, there is little epidemiologic data about second impact syndrome and its existence somewhat controversial [109]. One systematic review found 36 cases of second impact syndrome in the medical literature. It demonstrated that risk factors may include age 16–19 years old, participation in American football, and male gender [110]. There is currently no consensus on the length of time in between hits that an individual can suffer second impact syndrome; but if an athlete is still symptomatic, they may be at risk [111]. Cases of second impact syndrome that resulted in death have unsurprisingly garnered significant media attention and concern in many communities. As such, every state in the United States has adopted specific legislation regarding diagnosis and return to play following concussion to help protect athletes from returning to sport too quickly. Providers should become familiar with their respective state law with regards to concussion.

Chronic Traumatic Encephalopathy

Chronic traumatic encephalopathy (CTE) is a neurodegenerative condition that demonstrates deposition of tau proteins on autopsy. Therefore, it can only be diagnosed post-mortem. It is hypothesized to be caused by repetitive mild traumatic brain injuries or concussions. CTE has been described in former athletes with a history of concussion or repetitive head impact exposure, often accompanied by behavioral change [112]. Direct cause and effect has not been confirmed, though, making CTE a diagnosis that is currently widely debated. Advocates of CTE as a disease describe it as athletes presenting with behavioral disturbance, increased suicidality, and neurodegenerative disease leading to dementia [113]. A cause-and-effect relationship between post-mortem CTE changes and antemortem behavioral and cognitive manifestations has not been demonstrated yet. Many asymptomatic individuals have had confirmed CTE pathology at autopsy [114–116]. It is also unknown if CTE is a progressive disease and whether tau deposition is the cause of CTE or a byproduct or marker of a disease [117]. The incidence and prevalence of CTE in athletes and the general population also remain unknown, as brains are not routinely examined for CTE at autopsy [118].

CTE-associated symptoms may be related to numerous different factors. These include impact load and type, career length, genetic predisposition, or other lifestyle behaviors including alcohol, drug and anabolic steroid use, general health, and psychiatric disease [5]. Some retrospective studies have reported increased risk of neurodegenerative disease in former professional football players; however, former high school football players do not show a higher prevalence of neurodegenerative disease when compared to non-football peers [119, 120]. Concurrent extensive exposure to repetitive head impacts and number of diagnosed concussions is the most cited risk factor CTE, but the degree of exposure is likely specific to each individual, with multiple modifying risk factors [121]. A contact sport athlete or former athlete that presents with prolonged neuropsychiatric symptoms should be evaluated for potentially treatable comorbid conditions and not assumed to have CTE [122].

Suicidality

In recent years, there have been several prominent professional athletes that have committed suicide. Many of these cases have been hypothesized to be related to repetitive head injuries or CTE; however, no clear link has yet been established [123]. Depression is a clear risk factor for suicide, but underlying causes of depression in athletes and former athletes are likely multifactorial. A large number of retired National Football League (NFL) players have experienced difficulty adjusting to life after sports, trouble finding employment, financial struggles, chronic pain, and use of prescription pain killers [124, 125]. All of these factors, in addition to recurrent head injury, could contribute to depression symptoms. A recent systematic review found that there is evidence of some former athletes in contact, collision, and combat sports who suffer from depression later in life, and there may be an association between this and a history of multiple concussions [126, 127]. However, former athletes are not at an increased risk of death by suicide [128]. More prospective research is needed regarding the relationship between recurrent head injury and suicide in athletes. What is clear is that any individual who suffers from depression should be treated appropriately and monitored for warning signs of suicide, rather than assumed to have a progressive neurodegenerative disease [129].

Key Points
- The term persistent post-concussive symptoms (PPCS) is currently favored in the sports medicine community as it captures all patients who do not recover as anticipated following a concussion. Persisting symptoms after concussion (PSaC) is a newer term but is not yet widespread in the literature.
- The exact pathophysiology behind PPCS is unknown, but is likely multifactorial.
- Current evidence suggests that management of prolonged symptoms should focus on active treatment of specific primary and secondary diagnoses identified on assessment.
- Emerging evidence suggests that light exercise, rather than prolonged rest, is helpful in recovery from PPCS.

- Referrals should be considered for PPCS and guided toward specific symptoms, which may include neuropsychology/psychology, psychiatry, neurology, ophthalmology, optometry (vision/light therapy), sleep medicine, physical therapy, and occupational therapy.
- Second impact syndrome is a rare but catastrophic condition that could occur if an athlete is returned to activity prior to full recovery from a concussion.
- Long-term sequelae of repetitive concussions and PPCS are not clear but could include depression, anxiety, suicidality, and chronic traumatic encephalopathy (CTE).

References

1. American Psychiatric Association. Task force on DSM-IV. In: Diagnostic and statistical manual of mental disorders: DSM-IV-TR, vol. xxxvii. 4th ed. Washington: American Psychiatric Association; 2000. p. 943.
2. World Health Organization. The ICD-10 classification of mental and behavioural disorders: clinical descriptions and diagnostic guidelines, vol. xii. Geneva: World Health Organization; 1992. p. 362.
3. Reichenberg LW. DSM-5TM essentials: the savvy clinician's guide to the changes in criteria. Hoboken: Wiley; 2014.
4. McCrory P, Meeuwisse W, Dvorak J, Aubry M, Bailes J, Broglio S, et al. Consensus statement on concussion in sport-the 5(th) international conference on concussion in sport held in Berlin, October 2016. Br J Sports Med. 2017;51(11):838–47.
5. Harmon KG, Clugston JR, Dec K, Hainline B, Herring SA, Kane S, et al. American medical society for sports medicine position statement on concussion in sport. Clin J Sport Med. 2019;29(2):87–100.
6. Patricios JS, Schneider KJ, Dvorak J, Ahmed OH, Blauwet C, Cantu RC, et al. Consensus statement on concussion in sport: the 6th international conference on concussion in sport-Amsterdam, October 2022. Br J Sports Med. 2023;57(11):695–711.
7. McCrea M, Guskiewicz K, Randolph C, Barr WB, Hammeke TA, Marshall SW, et al. Incidence, clinical course, and predictors of prolonged recovery time following sport-related concussion in high school and college athletes. J Int Neuropsychol Soc. 2013;19(1):22–33.
8. Zemek R, Barrowman N, Freedman SB, Gravel J, Gagnon I, McGahern C, et al. Clinical risk score for persistent postconcussion symptoms among children with acute concussion in the ED. JAMA. 2016;315(10):1014–25.
9. Marshall CM, Vernon H, Leddy JJ, Baldwin BA. The role of the cervical spine in post-concussion syndrome. Phys Sportsmed. 2015;43(3):274–84.
10. Iverson GL, Gardner AJ, Terry DP, Ponsford JL, Sills AK, Broshek DK, et al. Predictors of clinical recovery from concussion: a systematic review. Br J Sports Med. 2017;51(12):941–8.
11. Fried E, Balla U, Catalogna M, Kozer E, Oren-Amit A, Hadanny A, et al. Persistent post-concussive syndrome in children after mild traumatic brain injury is prevalent and vastly underdiagnosed. Sci Rep. 2022;12(1):4364.
12. Romeu-Mejia R, Giza CC, Goldman JT. Concussion pathophysiology and injury biomechanics. Curr Rev Musculoskelet Med. 2019;
13. Clark CN, Edwards MJ, Ong BE, Goodliffe L, Ahmad H, Dilley MD, et al. Reframing post-concussional syndrome as an interface disorder of neurology, psychiatry and psychology. Brain. 2022;145(6):1906–15.

14. Ellis MJ, Leddy JJ, Willer B. Physiological, vestibulo-ocular and cervicogenic post-concussion disorders: an evidence-based classification system with directions for treatment. Brain Inj. 2015;29(2):238–48.

15. King ML, Lichtman SW, Seliger G, Ehert FA, Steinberg JS. Heart-rate variability in chronic traumatic brain injury. Brain Inj. 1997;11(6):445–53.

16. Hanna-Pladdy B, Berry ZM, Bennett T, Phillips HL, Gouvier WD. Stress as a diagnostic challenge for postconcussive symptoms: sequelae of mild traumatic brain injury or physiological stress response. Clin Neuropsychol. 2001;15(3):289–304.

17. Bakhtadze MA, Vernon H, Karalkin AV, Pasha SP, Tomashevskiy IO, Soave D. Cerebral perfusion in patients with chronic neck and upper back pain: preliminary observations. J Manipulative Physiol Ther. 2012;35(2):76–85.

18. Nakamura Y, Nojiri K, Yoshihara H, Takahata T, Honda-Takahashi K, Kubo S, et al. Significant differences of brain blood flow in patients with chronic low back pain and acute low back pain detected by brain SPECT. J Orthop Sci. 2014;19(3):384–9.

19. Freitag P, Greenlee MW, Wachter K, Ettlin TM, Radue EW. fMRI response during visual motion stimulation in patients with late whiplash syndrome. Neurorehabil Neural Repair. 2001;15(1):31–7.

20. Otte A, Mueller-Brand J, Fierz L. Brain SPECT findings in late whiplash syndrome. Lancet. 1995;345(8963):1513.

21. Alptekin K, Degirmenci B, Kivircik B, Durak H, Yemez B, Derebek E, et al. Tc-99m HMPAO brain perfusion SPECT in drug-free obsessive-compulsive patients without depression. Psychiatry Res. 2001;107(1):51–6.

22. Ito H, Kawashima R, Awata S, Ono S, Sato K, Goto R, et al. Hypoperfusion in the limbic system and prefrontal cortex in depression: SPECT with anatomic standardization technique. J Nucl Med. 1996;37(3):410–4.

23. Schwartz RB, Komaroff AL, Garada BM, Gleit M, Doolittle TH, Bates DW, et al. SPECT imaging of the brain: comparison of findings in patients with chronic fatigue syndrome, AIDS dementia complex, and major unipolar depression. AJR Am J Roentgenol. 1994;162(4):943–51.

24. Sarmento E, Moreira P, Brito C, Souza J, Jevoux C, Bigal M. Proton spectroscopy in patients with post-traumatic headache attributed to mild head injury. Headache. 2009;49(9):1345–52.

25. Bartnik-Olson BL, Holshouser B, Wang H, Grube M, Tong K, Wong V, et al. Impaired neurovascular unit function contributes to persistent symptoms after concussion: a pilot study. J Neurotrauma. 2014;31(17):1497–506.

26. Su SH, Xu W, Li M, Zhang L, Wu YF, Yu F, et al. Elevated C-reactive protein levels may be a predictor of persistent unfavourable symptoms in patients with mild traumatic brain injury: a preliminary study. Brain Behav Immun. 2014;38:111–7.

27. Rathbone AT, Tharmaradinam S, Jiang S, Rathbone MP, Kumbhare DA. A review of the neuro- and systemic inflammatory responses in post concussion symptoms: introduction of the "post-inflammatory brain syndrome" PIBS. Brain Behav Immun. 2015;46:1–16.

28. Meares S, Shores EA, Taylor AJ, Batchelor J, Bryant RA, Baguley IJ, et al. Mild traumatic brain injury does not predict acute postconcussion syndrome. J Neurol Neurosurg Psychiatry. 2008;79(3):300–6.

29. Clarke GJB, Skandsen T, Zetterberg H, Follestad T, Einarsen CE, Vik A, et al. Longitudinal associations between persistent post-concussion symptoms and blood biomarkers of inflammation and CNS-injury after mild traumatic brain injury. J Neurotrauma. 2024;41(7-8):862–78.

30. Lima Santos JP, Kontos AP, Mailliard S, Eagle SR, Holland CL, Suss SJ Jr, et al. White matter abnormalities associated with prolonged recovery in adolescents following concussion. Front Neurol. 2021;12:681467.

31. Lange RT, Iverson GL, Brubacher JR, Madler B, Heran MK. Diffusion tensor imaging findings are not strongly associated with postconcussional disorder 2 months following mild traumatic brain injury. J Head Trauma Rehabil. 2012;27(3):188–98.

32. Treleaven J, Jull G, Atkinson L. Cervical musculoskeletal dysfunction in post-concussional headache. Cephalalgia. 1994;14(4):273–9.
33. Jensen OK, Nielsen FF, Vosmar L. An open study comparing manual therapy with the use of cold packs in the treatment of post-traumatic headache. Cephalalgia. 1990;10(5):241–50.
34. Schneider KJ, Meeuwisse WH, Nettel-Aguirre A, Barlow K, Boyd L, Kang J, et al. Cervicovestibular rehabilitation in sport-related concussion: a randomised controlled trial. Br J Sports Med. 2014;48(17):1294–8.
35. Armstrong B, McNair P, Taylor D. Head and neck position sense. Sports Med. 2008;38(2):101–17.
36. Ernst A, Basta D, Seidl RO, Todt I, Scherer H, Clarke A. Management of posttraumatic vertigo. Otolaryngol Head Neck Surg. 2005;132(4):554–8.
37. Gard A, Al-Husseini A, Kornaropoulos EN, De Maio A, Tegner Y, Bjorkman-Burtscher I, et al. Post-concussive vestibular dysfunction is related to injury to the inferior vestibular nerve. J Neurotrauma. 2022;39(11-12):829–40.
38. Silverberg ND, Iverson GL. Etiology of the post-concussion syndrome: physiogenesis and psychogenesis revisited. Neuro Rehabil. 2011;29(4):317–29.
39. Iverson GL, Williams MW, Gardner AJ, Terry DP. Systematic review of preinjury mental health problems as a vulnerability factor for worse outcome after sport-related concussion. Orthop J Sports Med. 2020;8(10):2325967120950682.
40. Collins MW, Kontos AP, Reynolds E, Murawski CD, Fu FH. A comprehensive, targeted approach to the clinical care of athletes following sport-related concussion. Knee Surg Sports Traumatol Arthrosc. 2014;22(2):235–46.
41. Feddermann-Demont N, Echemendia RJ, Schneider KJ, Solomon GS, Hayden KA, Turner M, et al. What domains of clinical function should be assessed after sport-related concussion? A systematic review. Br J Sports Med. 2017;51(11):903–18.
42. Echemendia RJ, Brett BL, Broglio S, Davis GA, Giza CC, Guskiewicz KM, et al. Sport concussion assessment tool - 6 (SCAT6). Br J Sports Med. 2023;57(11):622–31.
43. Katz M, Lenoski S, Ali H, Craton N. Concussion office based rehabilitation assessment: a novel clinical tool for concussion assessment and management. Brain Sci. 2020;10(9)
44. Conder A, Conder R, Friesen C. Neurorehabilitation of persistent sport-related post-concussion syndrome. Neuro Rehabil. 2020;46(2):167–80.
45. McCrory P, Meeuwisse WH, Aubry M, Cantu RC, Dvorak J, Echemendia RJ, et al. Consensus statement on concussion in sport: the 4th international conference on concussion in sport, Zurich, November 2012. J Athl Train. 2013;48(4):554–75.
46. Makdissi M, Schneider KJ, Feddermann-Demont N, Guskiewicz KM, Hinds S, Leddy JJ, et al. Approach to investigation and treatment of persistent symptoms following sport-related concussion: a systematic review. Br J Sports Med. 2017;51(12):958–68.
47. Leddy JJ, Baker JG, Willer B. Active rehabilitation of concussion and post-concussion syndrome. Phys Med Rehabil Clin N Am. 2016;27(2):437–54.
48. Griesbach GS, Hovda DA, Molteni R, Wu A, Gomez-Pinilla F. Voluntary exercise following traumatic brain injury: brain-derived neurotrophic factor upregulation and recovery of function. Neuroscience. 2004;125(1):129–39.
49. Griesbach GS, Tio DL, Nair S, Hovda DA. Temperature and heart rate responses to exercise following mild traumatic brain injury. J Neurotrauma. 2013;30(4):281–91.
50. Darling SR, Leddy JJ, Baker JG, Williams AJ, Surace A, Miecznikowski JC, et al. Evaluation of the Zurich guidelines and exercise testing for return to play in adolescents following concussion. Clin J Sport Med. 2014;24(2):128–33.
51. Leddy JJ, Baker JG, Kozlowski K, Bisson L, Willer B. Reliability of a graded exercise test for assessing recovery from concussion. Clin J Sport Med. 2011;21(2):89–94.
52. Leddy JJ, Kozlowski K, Donnelly JP, Pendergast DR, Epstein LH, Willer B. A preliminary study of subsymptom threshold exercise training for refractory post-concussion syndrome. Clin J Sport Med. 2010;20(1):21–7.

53. Ellis MJ, Leddy J, Willer B. Multi-disciplinary management of athletes with post-concussion syndrome: an evolving pathophysiological approach. Front Neurol. 2016;7:136.
54. Leddy JJ, Haider MN, Ellis M, Willer BS. Exercise is medicine for concussion. Curr Sports Med Rep. 2018;17(8):262–70.
55. Silverberg ND, Iverson GL. Is rest after concussion "the best medicine?": recommendations for activity resumption following concussion in athletes, civilians, and military service members. J Head Trauma Rehabil. 2013;28(4):250–9.
56. Haider MN, Bezherano I, Wertheimer A, Siddiqui AH, Horn EC, Willer BS, et al. Exercise for sport-related concussion and persistent postconcussive symptoms. Sports Health. 2021;13(2):154–60.
57. Mucha A, Collins MW, Elbin RJ, Furman JM, Troutman-Enseki C, DeWolf RM, et al. A brief vestibular/ocular motor screening (VOMS) assessment to evaluate concussions: preliminary findings. Am J Sports Med. 2014;42(10):2479–86.
58. Ellis MJ, Cordingley D, Vis S, Reimer K, Leiter J, Russell K. Vestibulo-ocular dysfunction in pediatric sports-related concussion. J Neurosurg Pediatr. 2015;16(3):248–55.
59. Lau BC, Kontos AP, Collins MW, Mucha A, Lovell MR. Which on-field signs/symptoms predict protracted recovery from sport-related concussion among high school football players? Am J Sports Med. 2011;39(11):2311–8.
60. Collins MW, Kontos AP, Okonkwo DO, Almquist J, Bailes J, Barisa M, et al. Statements of agreement from the targeted evaluation and active management (TEAM) approaches to treating concussion meeting held in Pittsburgh, October 15-16, 2015. Neurosurgery. 2016;79(6):912–29.
61. Broglio SP, Collins MW, Williams RM, Mucha A, Kontos AP. Current and emerging rehabilitation for concussion: a review of the evidence. Clin Sports Med. 2015;34(2):213–31.
62. Hugentobler JA, Vegh M, Janiszewski B, Quatman-Yates C. Physical therapy intervention strategies for patients with prolonged mild traumatic brain injury symptoms: a case series. Int J Sports Phys Ther. 2015;10(5):676–89.
63. Ventura RE, Jancuska JM, Balcer LJ, Galetta SL. Diagnostic tests for concussion: is vision part of the puzzle? J Neuroophthalmol. 2015;35(1):73–81.
64. Gallaway M, Scheiman M, Mitchell GL. Vision therapy for post-concussion vision disorders. Optom Vis Sci. 2017;94(1):68–73.
65. Scheiman M, Cotter S, Kulp MT, Mitchell GL, Cooper J, Gallaway M, et al. Treatment of accommodative dysfunction in children: results from a randomized clinical trial. Optom Vis Sci. 2011;88(11):1343–52.
66. Thiagarajan P, Ciuffreda KJ. Effect of oculomotor rehabilitation on vergence responsivity in mild traumatic brain injury. J Rehabil Res Dev. 2013;50(9):1223–40.
67. LeMarshall SJ, Stevens LM, Ragg NP, Barnes L, Foster J, Canetti EFD. Virtual reality-based interventions for the rehabilitation of vestibular and balance impairments post-concussion: a scoping review. J Neuroeng Rehabil. 2023;20(1):31.
68. Raikes AC, Killgore WD. Potential for the development of light therapies in mild traumatic brain injury. Concussion. 2018;3(3):CNC57.
69. Bajaj S, Vanuk JR, Smith R, Dailey NS, Killgore WDS. Blue-light therapy following mild traumatic brain injury: effects on white matter water diffusion in the brain. Front Neurol. 2017;8:616.
70. Sinclair KL, Ponsford JL, Taffe J, Lockley SW, Rajaratnam SM. Randomized controlled trial of light therapy for fatigue following traumatic brain injury. Neurorehabil Neural Repair. 2014;28(4):303–13.
71. Ibrahim MM, Patwardhan A, Gilbraith KB, Moutal A, Yang X, Chew LA, et al. Long-lasting antinociceptive effects of green light in acute and chronic pain in rats. Pain. 2017;158(2):347–60.
72. Clark J, Hasselfeld K, Bigsby K, Divine J. Colored glasses to mitigate photophobia symptoms posttraumatic brain injury. J Athl Train. 2017;52(8):725–9.

73. Heslot C, Azouvi P, Perdrieau V, Granger A, Lefevre-Dognin C, Cogne M. A systematic review of treatments of post-concussion symptoms. J Clin Med. 2022;11(20)
74. Barth JT, Freeman JR, Broshek DK, Varney RN. Acceleration-deceleration sport-related concussion: the gravity of it all. J Athl Train. 2001;36(3):253–6.
75. Treleaven J. Dizziness, unsteadiness, visual disturbances, and postural control: implications for the transition to chronic symptoms after a whiplash trauma. Spine (Phila Pa 1976). 2011;36(25 Suppl):S211–7.
76. Schneider KJ, Iverson GL, Emery CA, McCrory P, Herring SA, Meeuwisse WH. The effects of rest and treatment following sport-related concussion: a systematic review of the literature. Br J Sports Med. 2013;47(5):304–7.
77. Seifert T. Post-traumatic headache therapy in the athlete. Curr Pain Headache Rep. 2016;20(6):41.
78. Cushman DM, Borowski L, Hansen C, Hendrick J, Bushman T, Teramoto M. Gabapentin and tricyclics in the treatment of post-concussive headache, a retrospective cohort study. Headache. 2019;59(3):371–82.
79. Pinto SM, Twichell MF, Henry LC. Predictors of pharmacological intervention in adolescents with protracted symptoms after sports-related concussion. PM R. 2017;9(9):847–55.
80. Stilling J, Paxman E, Mercier L, Gan LS, Wang M, Amoozegar F, et al. Treatment of persistent post-traumatic headache and post-concussion symptoms using repetitive transcranial magnetic stimulation: a pilot, double-blind, randomized controlled trial. J Neurotrauma. 2020;37(2):312–23.
81. Brooks BL, Sayers P, Virani S, Rajaram A, Tomfohr L. Insomnia in adolescents with slow recovery from concussion. J Neurotrauma. 2019;
82. Hoffman NL, Weber ML, Broglio SP, McCrea M, McAllister TW, Schmidt JD, et al. Influence of postconcussion sleep duration on concussion recovery in collegiate athletes. Clin J Sport Med. 2017;
83. Howell DR, Oldham JR, Brilliant AN, Meehan WP 3rd. Trouble falling asleep after concussion is associated with higher symptom burden among children and adolescents. J Child Neurol. 2019;34(5):256–61.
84. Oyegbile TO, Dougherty A, Tanveer S, Zecavati N, Delasobera BE. High sleep disturbance and longer concussion duration in repeat concussions. Behav Sleep Med. 2019:1–8.
85. Brent DA, Max J. Psychiatric sequelae of concussions. Curr Psychiatry Rep. 2017;19(12):108.
86. Vuletic S, Bell KR, Jain S, Bush N, Temkin N, Fann JR, et al. Telephone problem-solving treatment improves sleep quality in service members with combat-related mild traumatic brain injury: results from a randomized clinical trial. J Head Trauma Rehabil. 2016;31(2):147–57.
87. Theadom A, Barker-Collo S, Jones K, Dudley M, Vincent N, Feigin V. A pilot randomized controlled trial of on-line interventions to improve sleep quality in adults after mild or moderate traumatic brain injury. Clin Rehabil. 2018;32(5):619–29.
88. Ludwig R, Rippee M, D'Silva L, Radel J, Eakman AM, Beltramo A, et al. Cognitive behavioral therapy for insomnia improves sleep outcomes in individuals with concussion: a preliminary randomized wait-list control study. J Head Trauma Rehabil. 2024;
89. Killgore WDS, Vanuk JR, Shane BR, Weber M, Bajaj S. A randomized, double-blind, placebo-controlled trial of blue wavelength light exposure on sleep and recovery of brain structure, function, and cognition following mild traumatic brain injury. Neurobiol Dis. 2020;134:104679.
90. Raikes AC, Dailey NS, Shane BR, Forbeck B, Alkozei A, Killgore WDS. Daily morning blue light therapy improves daytime sleepiness, sleep quality, and quality of life following a mild traumatic brain injury. J Head Trauma Rehabil. 2020;35(5):E405–E21.
91. Trojian TH, Wang DH, Leddy JJ. Nutritional supplements for the treatment and prevention of sports-related concussion-evidence still lacking. Curr Sports Med Rep. 2017;16(4):247–55.
92. Barlow KM, Esser MJ, Veidt M, Boyd R. Melatonin as a treatment after traumatic brain injury: a systematic review and meta-analysis of the pre-clinical and clinical literature. J Neurotrauma. 2019;36(4):523–37.

93. Barlow KM, Brooks BL, Esser MJ, Kirton A, Mikrogianakis A, Zemek RL, et al. Efficacy of melatonin in children with postconcussive symptoms: a randomized clinical trial. Pediatrics. 2020;145(4)

94. Barlow KM, Kirk V, Brooks B, Esser MJ, Yeates KO, Zemek R, et al. Efficacy of melatonin for sleep disturbance in children with persistent post-concussion symptoms: secondary analysis of a randomized controlled trial. J Neurotrauma. 2021;38(8):950–9.

95. Howell DR, Potter MN, Provance AJ, Wilson PE, Kirkwood MW, Wilson JC. Sleep problems and melatonin prescription after concussion among youth athletes. Clin J Sport Med. 2021;31(6):475–80.

96. Lavigne G, Khoury S, Chauny JM, Desautels A. Pain and sleep in post-concussion/mild traumatic brain injury. Pain. 2015;156(Suppl 1):S75–85.

97. Roberts AL, Pascual-Leone A, Speizer FE, Zafonte RD, Baggish AL, Taylor H Jr, et al. Exposure to American football and neuropsychiatric health in former national football league players: findings from the football players health study. Am J Sports Med. 2019;47(12):2871–80.

98. Golding L, Gillingham RG, Perera NKP. The prevalence of depressive symptoms in high-performance athletes: a systematic review. Phys Sportsmed. 2020;48(3):247–58.

99. McCarty CA, Zatzick D, Stein E, Wang J, Hilt R, Rivara FP, et al. Collaborative care for adolescents with persistent postconcussive symptoms: a randomized trial. Pediatrics. 2016;138(4)

100. Mittenberg W, Canyock EM, Condit D, Patton C. Treatment of post-concussion syndrome following mild head injury. J Clin Exp Neuropsychol. 2001;23(6):829–36.

101. Al Sayegh A, Sandford D, Carson AJ. Psychological approaches to treatment of postconcussion syndrome: a systematic review. J Neurol Neurosurg Psychiatry. 2010;81(10):1128–34.

102. Whittaker R, Kemp S, House A. Illness perceptions and outcome in mild head injury: a longitudinal study. J Neurol Neurosurg Psychiatry. 2007;78(6):644–6.

103. Echemendia RJ, Gioia GA. The role of neuropsychologists in concussion evaluation and management. Handb Clin Neurol. 2018;158:179–91.

104. Silverberg ND, Panenka WJ. Antidepressants for depression after concussion and traumatic brain injury are still best practice. BMC Psychiatry. 2019;19(1):100.

105. McAllister TW, Zafonte R, Jain S, Flashman LA, George MS, Grant GA, et al. Randomized placebo-controlled trial of methylphenidate or galantamine for persistent emotional and cognitive symptoms associated with PTSD and/or traumatic brain injury. Neuropsychopharmacology. 2016;41(5):1191–8.

106. Johansson B, Wentzel AP, Andrell P, Mannheimer C, Ronnback L. Methylphenidate reduces mental fatigue and improves processing speed in persons suffered a traumatic brain injury. Brain Inj. 2015;29(6):758–65.

107. Quinn DK, Mayer AR, Master CL, Fann JR. Prolonged postconcussive symptoms. Am J Psychiatry. 2018;175(2):103–11.

108. Engelhardt J, Brauge D, Loiseau H. Second impact syndrome. Myth or reality? Neurochirurgie. 2021;67(3):265–75.

109. Bey T, Ostick B. Second impact syndrome. West J Emerg Med. 2009;10(1):6–10.

110. McLendon LA, Kralik SF, Grayson PA, Golomb MR. The controversial second impact syndrome: a review of the literature. Pediatr Neurol. 2016;62:9–17.

111. Weinstein E, Turner M, Kuzma BB, Feuer H. Second impact syndrome in football: new imaging and insights into a rare and devastating condition. J Neurosurg Pediatr. 2013;11(3):331–4.

112. McKee AC, Stern RA, Nowinski CJ, Stein TD, Alvarez VE, Daneshvar DH, et al. The spectrum of disease in chronic traumatic encephalopathy. Brain. 2013;136(Pt 1):43–64.

113. Randolph C. Chronic traumatic encephalopathy is not a real disease. Arch Clin Neuropsychol. 2018;33(5):644–8.

114. Iverson GL, Keene CD, Perry G, Castellani RJ. The need to separate chronic traumatic encephalopathy neuropathology from clinical features. J Alzheimers Dis. 2018;61(1):17–28.

115. McKee AC, Stein TD, Nowinski CJ, Stern RA, Daneshvar DH, Alvarez VE, et al. The spectrum of disease in chronic traumatic encephalopathy. Brain J Neurol. 2013;136(Pt 1):43–64.

116. Postupna N, Rose SE, Gibbons LE, Coleman NM, Hellstern LL, Ritchie K, et al. The delayed neuropathological consequences of traumatic brain injury in a community-based sample. Front Neurol. 2021;12:624696.
117. Stein TD, Alvarez VE, McKee AC. Chronic traumatic encephalopathy: a spectrum of neuropathological changes following repetitive brain trauma in athletes and military personnel. Alzheimers Res Ther. 2014;6(1):4.
118. Kelly JP, Priemer DS, Perl DP, Filley CM. Sports concussion and chronic traumatic encephalopathy: finding a path forward. Ann Neurol. 2023;93(2):222–5.
119. Savica R, Parisi JE, Wold LE, Josephs KA, Ahlskog JE. High school football and risk of neurodegeneration: a community-based study. Mayo Clin Proc. 2012;87(4):335–40.
120. Janssen PH, Mandrekar J, Mielke MM, Ahlskog JE, Boeve BF, Josephs K, et al. High school football and late-life risk of neurodegenerative syndromes, 1956-1970. Mayo Clin Proc. 2017;92(1):66–71.
121. Asken BM, Sullan MJ, DeKosky ST, Jaffee MS, Bauer RM. Research gaps and controversies in chronic traumatic encephalopathy: a review. JAMA Neurol. 2017;74(10):1255–62.
122. Asken BM, Sullan MJ, Snyder AR, Houck ZM, Bryant VE, Hizel LP, et al. Factors influencing clinical correlates of chronic traumatic encephalopathy (CTE): a review. Neuropsychol Rev. 2016;26(4):340–63.
123. Iverson GL. Suicide and chronic traumatic encephalopathy. J Neuropsychiatry Clin Neurosci. 2016;28(1):9–16.
124. Cottler LB, Ben Abdallah A, Cummings SM, Barr J, Banks R, Forchheimer R. Injury, pain, and prescription opioid use among former National Football League (NFL) players. Drug Alcohol Depend. 2011;116(1-3):188–94.
125. Schwenk TL, Gorenflo DW, Dopp RR, Hipple E. Depression and pain in retired professional football players. Med Sci Sports Exerc. 2007;39(4):599–605.
126. Manley G, Gardner AJ, Schneider KJ, Guskiewicz KM, Bailes J, Cantu RC, et al. A systematic review of potential long-term effects of sport-related concussion. Br J Sports Med. 2017;51(12):969–77.
127. Guskiewicz KM, Marshall SW, Bailes J, McCrea M, Harding HP Jr, Matthews A, et al. Recurrent concussion and risk of depression in retired professional football players. Med Sci Sports Exerc. 2007;39(6):903–9.
128. Lehman EJ, Hein MJ, Gersic CM. Suicide mortality among retired national football league players who played 5 or more seasons. Am J Sports Med. 2016;44(10):2486–91.
129. Iverson GL. Retired national football league players are not at greater risk for suicide. Arch Clin Neuropsychol. 2020;35(3):332–41.

Chapter 12
Concussion Prevention

Kathleen M. Weber, Daniel R. Kim, and Elizabeth B. Portin

Clinical Case

A mother and father accompany their 14-year-old son to his preseason pre-participation physical for high school sports. They inquire if there are any strategies or interventions that the high school is implementing to prevent concussions.

The following discussion will provide an overview of prevention strategies developed to reduce SRCs among athletes.

Protective Gear

Question: Are helmets effective at preventing concussions?

K. M. Weber (✉)
Rush University Medical Center, Midwest Orthopaedics at Rush, Chicago, IL, USA
e-mail: kathleen.weber@rushortho.com

D. R. Kim
Formally Rush University Sports Medicine Fellow, Meridian Sports Medicine Clinic, Anaheim, CA, USA

E. B. Portin
RUSH Pediatric Primary Care, Rush University Medical Center, Chicago, IL, USA
e-mail: Elizabeth_B_Portin@rush.edu

© The Author(s), under exclusive license to Springer Nature Switzerland AG 2025
D. S. Patel (ed.), *Concussion Management for Primary Care*,
https://doi.org/10.1007/978-3-031-85516-0_12

157

Helmets and Headgear

There is consensus among researchers, clinicians, and industry professionals that proper equipment, particularly helmets and headgear, protect against head injuries. The American Medical Society for Sports Medicine, for example, endorses helmet use to reduce scalp lacerations, skull fractures, and intracranial bleeds [1]. For a helmet or headgear to prevent an SRC, it must attenuate linear and rotational acceleration, which are the primary underlying mechanisms of SRCs [2].

Researchers have not been able to prove that helmets reduce SRCs, notwithstanding anecdotal evidence to the contrary. Investigating the effect of helmets to reduce SRC has proven to be challenging, especially in football, hockey, and other team collision sports, due to co-variability and ethical issues around having cohorts of athletes sustain from wearing helmets and comparing the rate of concussions in this group with athletes that are wearing helmets [3]. Players wear a variety of helmet brands and models, and different helmets may perform better under certain circumstances or when used by athletes in specific positions.

Changes to helmet design often involve tradeoffs. For example, heavier helmets typically attenuate linear acceleration but are less comfortable and accelerate rotational momentum and the duration of such rotation [2]. Many new helmet designs significantly reduce direct focal external force transfers, but these designs have not been proven to prevent linear and rotational acceleration. Interestingly, some argue that wearing seemingly more protective equipment, such as full-face masks in hockey and thicker padding in football helmets, may, in fact, increase risky behaviors in wearers stemming from a false sense of security thereby exposing them to a greater risk for SRCs and other injuries [1, 4].

Football

Question: Are there specific football helmets that prevent concussions?

Football helmet manufacturers have developed and continue to develop helmets incorporating new designs and materials intended to reduce SRCs. The National Football League (NFL), in conjunction with the National Football League Players Association, the NFL players' union, conducts an annual laboratory test, the NFL/NFLPA Helmet Performance Test, which simulates certain concussion-causing impacts to assess the performance of helmets worn by NFL players [5]. According to the 2022 NFL/NFLPA Helmet Performance Test press release, approximately 27% of returning players between the 2020 and 2021 seasons opted to switch to a better-performing helmet after reviewing the study's results and claim that adoption of such helmets has contributed to a 25% reduction in concussions among NFL players in 2018–2021 compared to 2015–2017 [5]. Nevertheless, research unaffiliated with the NFL has failed to show a meaningful difference in the incidence of SRCs with newer helmet models [6]. A 2023 meta-analysis reports mixed results among studies examining the effect of helmet type, padding thickness, and helmet lining on SRC rate [7].

Other Sports

Question: Should soccer or other sport athletes wear headgear to prevent concussions?

Studies have found that ski and snowboard helmets provide protection against head injuries, but, as another study pointed out, the studies did not separate concussions from other head injuries when looking at their efficacy toward concussion prevention [3, 8, 9]. Several bicycle helmets, especially newer designs, have built-in mechanisms to reduce rotational head acceleration caused by an oblique impact [10–12]. Wearing headgear in soccer has been explored with conflicting evidence for SRC reduction benefit, with a 2020 randomized controlled trial suggesting that headgear did not reduce the incidence or severity of SRC in high school soccer players [13, 14]. In the past, rugby headgear has not provided any protection against concussions [15]. However, newer headgear using a viscoelastic material has shown the ability to reduce linear and rotational impact energy in the test setting, which could potentially help reduce the rate of developing and the severity of concussions in rugby [16]. Again, it is unknown whether protective gear indirectly encourages higher risk behavior, and this possibility should be considered in discussions regarding changes to sport-specific headgear implementation.

Mouthguards

Question: Do mouthguards have any effect in preventing or reducing the severity of concussions?

It is widely accepted that mouthguards protect against overall head injury, especially dental injuries, while playing contact sports. However, the effectiveness of mouthguards in reducing the incidence or severity of concussions specifically is less clear [17, 18]. A meta-analysis did suggest that mouthguards protect against concussions in contact sports, specifically basketball, ice hockey, and rugby, but the findings were only statistically significant in ice hockey [7]. They found no difference in SRC protection between dentist fit mouthguards and off-the-shelf types [7]. The 2022 International Conference on Concussion in Sport's consensus statement recommends mouthguard use in child and adolescent ice hockey [19].

Neck Compression Collars

Question: Do neck compression collars have any effect in preventing or reducing the severity of concussions?

A neck compression device known as the Q-Collar has been cleared by the FDA in 2021 to aid in the protection of the brain from the effects associated with repetitive sub-concussive head impacts [20]. It is a C-shaped collar purported to apply slight compression to the jugular veins and increase blood volume in the cranial space and reduce movement of the brain during impact. While it has been demonstrated to be safe, evidence regarding neurologic benefit is limited to MRI and fMRI studies that show differences in the diffusion and anisotropic properties of brain white matter comparing collared and non-collared high school athletes who had similar levels of head trauma [21–23]. However, there is currently no empirical evidence that it reduces the risk of concussion, serious head injury, or decline in demonstrated cognitive ability.

Fit and Maintenance

Question: Are there any reputable sources to assist with the proper fit of headgear?

Ensuring the proper fit of equipment is paramount. The use of an ill-fitting helmet, for example, is a risk factor for concussions with more symptoms and of longer duration [7, 24]. The Centers for Disease Control launched a mobile web-based application as part of their larger Heads Up: Concussion program to help find a properly fitting helmet for various sports [25]. It is also important to periodically inspect helmets, mouthguards, and other equipment throughout sports seasons in addition to at the beginning of each season and to repair or replace whatever has become deformed, worn down, or ill-fitting [24]. Moreover, designating a specific person to monitor for proper fit is essential, especially in youth and high school athletes where head size and hairstyle may change throughout the season.

Cost

Unfortunately, protective equipment in contact sports can be expensive. In 2016, the Gadsden Times, an Alabama newspaper, estimated that the cost of outfitting a high school football player for a practice and a game might be between $800 and $1000 [26]. The list price of the top-ranked helmet in the 2024 NFL/NFLPA Helmet Performance Test is roughly $1200 [27].

Such expenses typically present, at minimum, financial hardship to parents and/ or school districts and may even bar youth participation in the sport altogether. Programs that help provide youth athletes or youth sports teams with new or gently used equipment, such as Good Sports [28], Sports Matter [29], and The Sports Shed [30], may help reduce these costs. Additional care is required to ensure that such equipment is appropriate and fits correctly [31].

Athlete Bias

Question: Do athletes use the safety-related equipment that is designed to reduce the risk of concussion?

Countless examples exist of professional athletes resisting safety-related equipment upgrades for behavioral and even cosmetic reasons [32, 33]. For example, the overwhelming majority of Major League Baseball pitchers do not wear protective liners and caps designed to protect them from dangerous line drives hit back at them. Such intransigence has been addressed through a combination of rule changes at professional and youth levels designed to socialize these players from a young age to the more protective equipment [34].

Technique

Question: Are sports organizations incorporating skill instruction in an attempt to reduce the risk of sports-related concussions?

More than ever, organized sports have largely replaced neighborhood pickup games beloved by previous generations of Americans. While the proliferation of organized sport has its detractors and disadvantages, one potential benefit is an increase in opportunities for youth participants to learn proper techniques, especially in high-risk maneuvers associated with SRCs, such as football tackling, hockey body-checking and soccer heading [1, 35, 36].

Using this time for skill development and instruction instead of games may reduce SRCs. Athletes learn better body control to prepare them for the inevitable collisions that will occur when they grow older and join leagues that permit these maneuvers. This training now incorporates sport-specific techniques to reduce head acceleration.

Football

USA Football, a youth football governing body, heavily promotes Heads Up Football (HUF), a series of online and in-person courses for coaches to learn about proper equipment fitting, tackling technique and drills designed to reduce head contact [37]. HUF's tackling module includes fundamentals of and systems for teaching shoulder tackling and draws on principles of rugby tackling, which does not use the head [38]. A 2015 study found that HUF reduced injury rates, but the New York Times raised issues with how USA Football and the study's authors presented certain data from that study [35, 39, 40]. Further, that study evaluated the entire HUF program, so the efficacy, if any, of the HUF tackling model on reducing SRCs is unknown.

Soccer

Strategies to reduce head acceleration when heading the ball in soccer include achieving head-neck-torso alignment and neck strengthening (discussed below) [41, 42]. Other experts recommend using lightweight soccer balls to teach and perfect heading techniques [42]. In theory these recommendations make sense but lack the support of strong evidence based clinical research.

Hockey

Coaching and education programs in the United States and Canada emphasize teaching youth to keep their heads up, especially when about to receive a check. Since the implementation of programs emphasizing these skills, there has been a decrease in cervical spine injuries, but the effectiveness of these techniques have not been formally assessed [43]. USA Hockey's American Development model emphasizes skill and skating development including proper body control, angling, and body contact but does not teach body-checking skills until 11- to 12-year-old age group [43].

Neck Strengthening

Question: Do neck strengthening exercises prevent concussions?

Small and/or weak neck musculature is an SRC's risk factor [44]. Neck strengthening may help prevent SRCs by reducing head acceleration [45, 46]. Support for neck strengthening exists primarily based on anecdotal evidence and lab-based testing, but clinical evidence is mixed with regards to neck strength, endurance, or circumference as a modifiable risk factor for SRC risk according to a 2023 meta-analysis [7]. One study found that every 1-pound increase in neck strength contributes to a 5% decrease in odds for a concussive event to occur [44]. This protective benefit is likely due to the decreased kinematic response of the head to controlled impulsive loading with greater neck strength [45]. Another study reported a 13% lower rate of SRC for every 10% increase in neck extension strength in professional rugby players, but other neck strength measures including a composite measure were not significantly associated with SRC. Two other studies did not support the above findings and did not find any association with collegiate athletes' SRC risk and preseason deep neck flexor endurance or neck circumference measures [47, 48]. It is also believed that neck-strengthening exercises are more likely to reduce SRCs in females than males due to females' weaker necks [1, 44, 49–52]. Multiple neck strengthening programs have been proposed that show promise [45, 53]. However, further research is required on the benefit of neck strengthening on concussion prevention during actual play.

Supplementation

Question: Can supplements play a role in concussion management?

There is currently no strong evidence to support the use of supplements for concussion prevention or treatment. However, there have been preclinical studies showing promising results regarding various supplements. Omega-3 fatty acids (O3FA) have been shown to decrease markers of oxidative stress and normalize modulators of neuronal plasticity in animal studies [54], but there is no strong clinical evidence in humans. Similarly, neuroprotective findings in animal studies are reported for curcumin and melatonin, while creatine and vitamins C, D, and E have shown utility in the use of severe brain trauma with no direct research on their use in concussions [55]. As human trials are underway, supplements may play a role in the prevention and/or treatment of concussions in the future, but currently the evidence does not support their use.

Rule Changes

Question: How effective have rule changes been in reducing the number of concussions? Is there a difference in the effectiveness from sport to sport?

Rule changes intended to reduce collisions that often result in concussion have been proposed and implemented in several sports. The difficulty in coming up with new rules is finding a balance between limiting the number of head collisions while maintaining the game's integrity. Additionally, rule changes in specific sports cannot be generally applied across all levels of play from youth to the elite level.

Football

Football has implemented several safety-related rule changes in an effort to reduce SRCs and other injuries. In 2011, the NFL moved the kickoff line forward by five yards in an attempt to prevent concussions. That rule change was intended to increase rates of touchbacks on kickoffs, a play involving high-speed collisions in which a disproportionate number of SRCs have been found to occur. In 2016, the Ivy League, a Division I National Collegiate Athletic Association conference, moved the kickoff and touchback lines up to the 40-yard and 25-yard lines, respectively, for the same reasons. A 2018 study found these rule changes reduce the average annual concussion rate in Ivy League football by more than 68% [56].

Certain youth football leagues have postponed tackling until a certain age and/or reduced the number of contact practices [57]. The NFL also adopted a rule beginning in the 2018–2019 season making it a foul for a player to lower his head to initiate and make contact with his helmet against an opponent [58]. In 2023, the NFL made it a foul for players to use their helmet to "butt, ram, spear" or make forcible contact to opponents' head or neck area in any way [59].

Hockey

Body-checking and fighting, which are associated with higher risk of SRCs, are hot button, safety-related issues debated in hockey. Until the 2010–2011 season, a body check to an opponent's head as the primary point of contact was legal in the National Hockey League (NHL). Beginning that season, in an effort to prevent SRCs and other head injuries, the NHL adopted Rule 48.1, which made *targeting* an opponent's head from the blind side illegal. An independent study released in July 2013 found no decrease in concussion incidence among NHL players following implementation of Rule 48 [1, 60].

Removing body-checking at the youth level has also gained popularity [43]. Since 2011, USA Hockey, the American youth hockey governing board, has prohibited all body-checking in players 12 and younger [43]. In Canada, the age at which body-checking is allowed has also increased to 13 years old [43]. A 2011 Canadian study found that eliminating body-checking under age 13 led to significant reduction in SRCs among youth 13 and under compared to SRCs among similarly aged youth playing in leagues that allowed checking [61]. Opponents of the youth body-checking ban were concerned that such a ban would increase the risk of injury, including SRCs, to young players by depriving them of the chance to learn proper body-checking technique once they grew and joined leagues in which body-checking is permissible. The authors of this chapter are not aware of any research that substantiates this concern, and the same 2011 Canadian study specifically refuted it [43, 61]. Disallowing body-checking has also been incorporated into older age groups in non-elite levels, but the impact on concussions in these groups requires further investigation [62].

In an effort to reduce fighting, beginning the 2016–2017 season, the American Hockey League adopted Rule 23.7, which provides an automatic one-game suspension after a player incurs ten fighting major penalties during the regular season [63]. The Ontario Hockey League adopted a similar rule in 2011 [64].

Other Sports

Other sports have also instituted rule changes in an effort to reduce SRCs. For example, since 2014, Major League Baseball has banned avoidable collisions between catchers and base runners at home plate by initiating a rule that disallows runners attempting to score from deviating from his direct pathway to the plate and the catcher is not permitted to block the runner's path to the plate unless he is in possession of the ball [65]. Green et al. found that this rule change was associated with significant reductions in the numbers of concussions and other injuries cause by collisions at home plate [66]. In 2015, US Soccer, the soccer governing body in the United States, banned heading among players younger than age 10 and limited the amount of heading in practice among players ages 11–13 [67, 68].

Rule Enforcement

Question: How effective have rule changes been in reducing illegal play?

While the rules of play form the basis of safer play, athletes, coaches, and officials need to adhere to the rules in order for them to make a difference [43]. In high school athletes, illegal activity contributed to over 10% of injuries in boys' and girls' soccer and basketball, and concussions made up the greatest percentage of those injuries [69]. The injuries related to illegal play are even greater in other leagues and have been reported to be as high as 50% [69, 70]. Promoting fair and safer play requires an attitude shift and modeling by coaches, parents, officials, and managers in addition to the athletes. In ice hockey, Fair Play rules, a program developed to reward teams with good sportsmanship, has contributed to a significant reduction in injuries including concussions [43]. Additionally, the zero tolerance to head contact rule change in the NHL has led to a 36% reduction in concussion risk [60]. In soccer, stricter enforcement of red cards for high elbows during heading duals has led to a slightly reduced risk of concussion [3, 71].

Legislation

Question: Have states implemented legislation to protect children from SRCs? Is medical clearance needed prior to returning to sports following a concussion?

Concussion management in youth sports is subject to a state-by-state patchwork of laws and regulations [72, 73]. The most well-known of these laws is Washington State's Lystedt Law [74]. The Lystedt Law was enacted in 2009 in the aftermath of the tragic death of Zackery Lystedt who suffered multiple concussions in a single game resulting in intracranial hemorrhage and severe traumatic brain injury. The Lystedt Law has three main components: [1] removal, [2] medical clearance for return-to-play, and [3] education [72, 74]. Since the Lystedt Law's enactment, all 50 states have enacted some form of legislation to protect children from SRCs. Many of these are patterned on the Lystedt Law but significant differences exist.

Several studies have looked at the impact of the Lystedt Law in Washington State and similar laws in other states on concussions in high school athletes [73, 75–77]. Studies have found an increase both in the frequency of concussions and the mean number of days during which concussed youths are held out of play. This is likely due to the increased awareness of concussions in addition to the need for medical clearance prior to returning to play. In regard to implementation, high school football and soccer coaches in Washington State endorsed receiving appropriate concussion education 3 years after the Lystedt Law was passed [78]. However, there is still a lot that must be done to in regard to implementation of the laws. One study found that after enacting a concussion law in Ohio the rate of follow-up after an initial ED visit for concussion increased from 44% prelaw to 58% post-law, which means that nearly 40% of concussed players did not receive appropriate follow-up and therefore clearance [73, 76].

Education

Question: Do formal concussion education programs improve concussion knowledge? Does education decrease the rate of concussions?

Several formal education programs have been established that focus on both primary and secondary prevention strategies with specific information geared toward the athletes, coaches/staff, parents, healthcare providers, and/or the public. There is consensus among policies, guidelines, and consensus statements on school sport injury prevention that education is the mainstay of concussion prevention [31]. A large component of programs is teaching improved identification and reporting of concussions to protect against athletes the potential consequences of playing with concussions. Most also emphasize strict adherence to return to play guidelines (refer to chapter on return to play). Programs also aim to educate on the short- and long-term consequences of suffering a concussion with the hope of changing attitudes on the playing field to prevent risky behaviors that may lead to concussions. Two studies examining child and adolescent American football players demonstrated that players exposed to a comprehensive coach education program had significantly lower practice-related head impacts and game and practice-related concussion rates relative to players in leagues that did not participate [35, 79]. The specific education method or program should be tailored to each individual group to optimize learning. Table 12.1 lists several education programs and resources that currently exist.

The annual pre-participation physical exam (PPE) can be very useful in identifying athletes who have a history of concussion and who may be at increased risk for concussion due to involvement in contact sports. The PPE provides an excellent educative opportunity to inform athletes and their parents of the significance of concussions [62]. The medical professional performing the exam should ask

Table 12.1 Concussion education programs and resources

Program	Target audience	Website
Barrow Brainbook	High school athletes	https://concussion.barrowneuro.org
Brain 101: The Concussion Playbook	Coaches Educators Parents Teen athletes	http://brain101.orcasinc.com/1000/
Concussion Legacy Foundation Team Up against Concussions Advanced Concussion Training	Schools, community centers, and athletic programs with youth in grades 4–12 Families, coaches, teachers, medical professionals, and athletes beyond high school	https://concussionfoundation.org/programs/education
The Center for Disease Control and Prevention's Heads Up	Coaches Parents Athletes School professionals Healthcare provider	www.cdc.gov/headsup/index.html
Heads Up Football	Coaches	usafootball.com/programs/heads-up-football/
National Federation of State High School Associations' Concussion for Students	High school athletes	https://nfhslearn.com/courses?searchText=Concussion
NCAA Concussion Educational Resources	College athletes Coaches Athletic trainers Team physicians Athletic directors	http://www.ncaa.org/sport-science-institute/concussion-educational-resources
Rugbysmart	Coaches Referees	www.rugbysmart.co.nz
ThinkFirst About Concussion	Youth and teens	http://thinkfirst.org/concussion

Note: This table is not exhaustive

concussion-related questions including past history of concussion, duration of symptoms, and the presence of mood, learning attention, or migraine disorders, which have been shown to complicate the diagnosis and management athletes [1]. However, there is no evidence that preexisting mood or learning disorders predispose athletes to concussions.

Conclusion

Researchers have made considerable progress over the past 20 or so years in determining the causes of SRCs but have made fewer inroads in determining how to prevent them. There is no cure-all to prevent SRCs. This much is known.

Nevertheless, much of the existing research is imprecise and/or unsatisfying and questions abound. More research is required, and until such research becomes available, PCPs are left to endorse SRC prevention strategies based largely on intuition and anecdotal evidence.

Key Points
- Investigating the effect of helmets to reduce SRC has proven to be challenging and requires on-going research.
- Teaching proper technique in sports activities such as sport-specific techniques to reduce head acceleration may help to reduce concussions.
- Rule changes intended to reduce collisions that often result in concussion have been proposed and implemented in several sports.
- More research is required, and until such research becomes available, PCPs are left to endorse SRC prevention strategies based largely on intuition and anecdotal evidence.

References

1. Harmon KG, Drezner JA, Gammons M. American medical society for sports medicine position statement: Concussion in sport. Br J Sports Med. 2013;47(1):15–26.
2. Zuckerman SL, Reynolds BB, Yengo-Kahn AM. A football helmet prototype that reduces linear and rotational acceleration with the addition of an outer shell. J Neurosurg. 2018:1–8.
3. Emery CA, Black AM, Kolstad A. What strategies can be used to effectively reduce the risk of concussion in sport? A systematic review. Br J Sports Med. 2017;51(12):978–84.
4. Schneider DK, Grandhi RK, Bansal P. Current state of concussion prevention strategies: a systematic review and meta-analysis of prospective, controlled studies. Br J Sports Med. 2017;51(20):1473–82.
5. NFL.com 2024. Unprecedented Rate Of Improvement Stimulated In Helmet Industry, New Standard Set For 'Top-Performing' Helmet Models Worn By NFL Players. Available from: https://www.nfl.com/playerhealthandsafety/resources/press-releases/unprecedented-rate-of-improvement-stimulated-in-helmet-industry-new-standard-set

6. McGuine TA, Hetzel S, McCrea M, Brooks MA. Protective equipment and player characteristics associated with the incidence of sport-related concussion in high school football players. Am J Sports Med. 2014;42(10):2470–8.
7. Eliason PH, Galarneau JM, Kolstad AT, Pankow MP, West SW, Bailey S, et al. Prevention strategies and modifiable risk factors for sport-related concussions and head impacts: a systematic review and meta-analysis. Br J Sports Med. 2023;57(12):749–61.
8. Haider AH, Saleem T, Bilaniuk JW, Barraco RD. An evidence-based review: efficacy of safety helmets in the reduction of head injuries in recreational skiers and snowboarders. J Trauma Acute Care Surgery. 2012;73(5):1340–7.
9. Hagel BE, Pless IB, Goulet C, Platt RW, Robitaille Y. Effectiveness of helmets in skiers and snowboarders: case-control and case crossover study. BMJ. 2005;330(7486):281–3.
10. Rowson S, Duma SM, Greenwald RM. Can helmet design reduce the risk of concussion in football? J Neurosurg. 2014;120(4):919–22.
11. Bland ML, Zuby DS, Mueller BC, Rowson S. Differences in the protective capabilities of bicycle helmets in real-world and standard-specified impact scenarios. Traffic Inj Prev. 2018;19(sup1)
12. Bland ML, McNally C, Rowson S. Differences in impact performance of bicycle helmets during oblique impacts. J Biomech Eng. 2018;140(9)
13. Delaney JS, Al-Kashmiri A, Drummond R, Correa JA. The effect of protective headgear on head injuries and concussions in adolescent football (soccer) players. Br J Sports Med. 2008;42(2):5.
14. McGuine T, Post E, Pfaller AY, Hetzel S, Schwarz A, Brooks MA, et al. Does soccer headgear reduce the incidence of sport-related concussion? A cluster, randomised controlled trial of adolescent athletes. Br J Sports Med. 2020;54(7):408–13.
15. Barnes A, Rumbold JL, Olusoga P. Attitudes towards protective headgear in UK rugby union players. BMJ Open Sport Exerc Med. 2017;3(1)
16. Ganly M, McMahon JM. New generation of headgear for rugby: impact reduction of linear and rotational forces by a viscoelastic material-based rugby head guard. BMJ Open Sport Exerc Med. 2018;4(1)
17. Harmon KG, Clugston DJR, K. American medical society for sports medicine position statement on concussion in sport. Br J Sports Med. 2019;53(4):213–25.
18. Halstead ME, Walter KD, Moffatt K. Sport-related concussion in children and adolescents. Pediatrics. 2018;142(6)
19. Patricios JS, Schneider KJ, Dvorak J, Ahmed OH, Blauwet C, Cantu RC, et al. Consensus statement on concussion in sport: the 6th international conference on concussion in sport-Amsterdam, October 2022. Br J Sports Med. 2023;57(11):695–711.
20. Commissioner O of the. FDA. FDA; 2021. FDA Authorizes Marketing of Novel Device to Help Protect Athletes' Brains During Head Impacts. Available from: https://www.fda.gov/news-events/press-announcements/fda-authorizes-marketing-novel-device-help-protect-athletes-brains-during-head-impacts
21. Diekfuss JA, Yuan W, Barber Foss KD, Dudley JA, DiCesare CA, Reddington DL, et al. The effects of internal jugular vein compression for modulating and preserving white matter following a season of American tackle football: a prospective longitudinal evaluation of differential head impact exposure. J Neurosci Res. 2021;99(2):423–45.
22. Yuan W, Dudley J, Barber Foss KD, Ellis JD, Thomas S, Galloway RT, et al. Mild jugular compression collar ameliorated changes in brain activation of working memory after one soccer season in female high school athletes. J Neurotrauma. 2018;35(11):1248–59.
23. Myer GD, Yuan W, Barber Foss KD, Thomas S, Smith D, Leach J, et al. Analysis of head impact exposure and brain microstructure response in a season-long application of a jugular vein compression collar: a prospective, neuroimaging investigation in American football. Br J Sports Med. 2016;50(20):1276–85.

24. Greenhill DA, Navo P, Zhao H, Torg J, Comstock RD, Boden BP. Inadequate helmet fit increases concussion severity in american high school football players. Sports Health Multidisciplinary Approach. 2016;8(3):238–43.
25. Centers for Disease Control and Prevention. CDC HEADS UP concussion and helmet safety.
26. Taylor K. The cost of high school football – dollars must be stretched to train, equip, feed teams. Gadsden Times. 2016;08(17) Available from: https://www.gadsdentimes.com/news/20160817/cost-of-high-school-football%2D%2D-dollars-must-be-stretched-to-train-equip-feed-teams
27. NFL.com 2024. Helmet Laboratory Testing Performance Results. Available from: https://www.nfl.com/playerhealthandsafety/equipment-and-innovation/equipment-testing/helmet-laboratory-testing-performance-results
28. Good Sports. Available from: https://www.goodsports.org/about/
29. Sports Matter: Help Save Youth Sports. Available from: https://www.sportsmatter.org
30. The Sports Shed. Available from: https://thesportsshed.org
31. Göpfert A, Hove M, Emond A, Mytton J. Prevention of sports injuries in children at school: a systematic review of policies. BMJ Open Sport Exerc Med. 2018;4(1)
32. Waldstein D. Safer batting helmet draws resistance from some players. New York Times August. 2009;12. Available from: https://www.nytimes.com/2009/08/13/sports/baseball/13helmet.html
33. Maske M. NFL players, including tom brady, will have to be in approved helmets this season [Internet]. Available from: https://search.proquest.com/docview/2208587151
34. NHL BM. NHLPA agree on mandatory visors. Available from: https://www.nhl.com/news/nhl-nhlpa-agree-on-mandatory-visors/c-672983
35. Kerr ZY, Yeargin S, Valovich McLeod TC. Comprehensive coach education and practice contact restriction guidelines result in lower injury rates in youth american football. Orthop. J Sports Med. 2015;3(7)
36. Kerr ZY, Dalton SL, Roos KG, Djoko A, Phelps J, Dompier TP. Comparison of indiana high school football injury rates by inclusion of the USA football "heads up football" player safety coach. Orthop J Sports Med. 2016;4(5)
37. Football USA. Heads up football
38. Schussler E, Jagacinski RJ, White SE, Chaudhari AM, Buford JA, Onate JA. The effect of tackling training on head accelerations in youth american football. Int J Sports Phys Ther. 2018;13(2):229–37.
39. SCHWARZ ALAN. N.F.L.-backed youth program says it reduced concussions the data disagrees [Internet]. Available from: https://search.proquest.com/docview/1807059662
40. Hallenbeck S. USA football statement on New York times article about heads up football. 2016.
41. Shewchenko N, Withnall C, Keown M, Gittens R, Dvorak J. Heading in football. Part 3: effect of ball properties on head response. Br J Sports Med. 2005;39(suppl 1)
42. Caccese J, Kaminski T. Minimizing head acceleration in soccer: a review of the literature. Sports Med. 2016;46(11):1591–604.
43. Anonymous. Reducing injury risk from body checking in boys' youth ice hockey. Pediatrics. 2014;133(6):1151–7.
44. Collins C, Fletcher E, Fields S. Neck strength: a protective factor reducing risk for concussion in high school sports. J Prim Prev. 2014;35(5):309–19.
45. Eckner JT, Goshtasbi A, Curtis K. Feasibility and effect of cervical resistance training on head kinematics in youth athletes: a pilot study. Am J Phys Med Rehabil. 2018;97(4):292–7.
46. Tierney RT, Higgins M, Caswell SV. Sex differences in head acceleration during heading while wearing soccer headgear. J Athl Train. 2008;43(6):578–84.
47. Baker M, Quesnele J, Baldisera T, Kenrick-Rochon S, Laurence M, Grenier S. Exploring the role of cervical spine endurance as a predictor of concussion risk and recovery following sports related concussion. Musculoskelet Sci Pract. 2019;42:193–7.
48. Esopenko C, De Souza N, Conway F, Todaro SM, Brostrand K, Womack J, et al. Bigger necks are not enough: an examination of neck circumference in incoming college athletes. J Prim Prev. 2020;41(5):421–9.

49. Benson BW, Gunter FE, Rauch R. What are the most effective risk-reduction strategies in sport concussion? J Med Genet. 2013;47(5)
50. Swanik KA, Tierney RT, Swanik CB, Sitler MR, Torg J, Higgins M. Gender differences in head-neck segment dynamics stabilization during head acceleration. Med Sci Sports Exerc. 2005;37(2)
51. Mansell J, Tierney RT, Sitler MR, Swanik KA, Stearne D. Resistance training and head-neck segment dynamic stabilization in male and female collegiate soccer players. J Athl Train. 2005;40(4)
52. Hildenbrand K, Vasavada A. Collegiate and high school athlete neck strength in neutral and rotated postures. J Strength Cond Res. 2013;27(11):3173–82.
53. Toninato J, et al. Traumatic brain injury reduction in athletes by neck strengthening (TRAIN). Contemp Clin Trials Commun. 2018;11:102–6.
54. Wu A, Ying Z, Gomez-Pinilla F. Dietary omega-3 fatty acids normalize BDNF levels, reduce oxidative damage, and counteract learning disability after traumatic brain injury in rats. J Neurotrauma. 2004;21(10):1457–67.
55. Ashbaugh A, McGrew C. The role of nutritional supplements in sports concussion treatment. Curr Sports Med Rep. 2016;15(1):16–9.
56. Wiebe DJ, D'Alonzo BA, Harris R, Putukian M, Campbell-McGovern C. Association between the experimental kickoff rule and concussion rates in ivy league football. JAMA. 2018;320(19)
57. Warner P. Limited Contact in Practice Rule. Available from: https://tshq.bluesombrero.com/Default.aspx?tabid=1476228
58. Use of the Helmet – Rule 12, Section 2, Article 8. Available from: https://nflcommunications.com/Documents/Fact%20Sheet%20-%20Use%20of%20the%20Helmet.pdf
59. NFL.com 2024. NFL Health and Safety Related Rules Changes Since 2002. Available from: https://www.nfl.com/playerhealthandsafety/equipment-and-innovation/rules-changes/nfl-health-and-safety-related-rules-changes-since-2002
60. Donaldson L, Asbridge M, Cusimano MD. Bodychecking rules and concussion in elite hockey. PLoS One. 2013;8(7)
61. Emery C, Kang J, Shrier I. Risk of injury associated with bodychecking experience among youth hockey players. CMAJ. 2011;183(11):1249–56.
62. McCrory P, Meeuwisse W, Dvořák J. Consensus statement on concussion in sport – the 5th international conference on concussion in sport held in berlin. Br J Sports Med. 2016;51(11):838.
63. American Hockey League Official Rule Book 2018-2019. Available from: https://theahl.com/rules
64. OHL Announces Player Safety Initiatives and Rule Changes for 2016-17 Season. Available from: http://ontariohockeyleague.com/article/ohl-announces-player-safety-initiatives-and-rule-changes-for-2016-17-season
65. Official Baseball Rules_2019 Official Baseball Rules 3/26/2019 5:16 PM Page i. In: 2019 official baseball Rules_2019 official baseball rules 3/26/2019 5:16 PM. 2019.
66. Green G, D'Angelo J, Coyles J, Penny I, Golfinos JG, Valadka A. Association between a rule change to reduce home plate collisions and mild traumatic brain injury and other injuries in professional baseball players. Am J Sports Med. 2019;47(11):2704–8.
67. U.S. Available from: https://www.ussoccer.com/about/recognize-to-recover/concussion-guidelines
68. Player Safety Campaign FAQs – US soccer . Available from: https://www.ussoccer.com/about/recognize-to-recover/concussion-guidelines/player-safety-campaign-faqs
69. Collins CL, Fields SK, Comstock RD. When the rules of the game are broken: what proportion of high school sports-related injuries are related to illegal activity? Inj Prev. 2008;14(1):34–8.
70. Junge A, Dvorak J, Graf-Baumann T, Peterson L. Football injuries during FIFA tournaments and the olympic games, 1998-2001. Am J Sports Med. 2004;32(1_suppl):80–9.
71. Bjørneboe J, Bahr R, Dvorak J, Andersen TE. Lower incidence of arm-to-head contact incidents with stricter interpretation of the laws of the game in norwegian male professional football. Br J Sports Med. 2013;47(8):508–14.

72. Spaude LK. Time to act: correcting the inadequacy of youth concussion legislation through a federal act. Marquette Law Rev. 2017;100(3)
73. Fisher PG. Have zackery lystedt concussion laws made an impact? J Pediatr. 2019;206:2–3.
74. Chapter 4, Laws of 2. Engrossed house bill 1824.
75. Davies S, Coxe K, Harvey HH, Singichetti B, Guo J, Yang J. Qualitative evaluation of high school implementation strategies for youth sports concussion laws. J Athl Train. 2018;53(9):873–9.
76. Tarimala A, Singichetti B, Yi H. Initial emergency department visit and follow-up care for concussions among children with medicaid. J Pediatr. 2019;206:178–83.
77. Bompadre V, Jinguji TM, Yanez ND. Washington state's lystedt law in concussion documentation in seattle public high schools. J Athl Train. 2014;49(4)
78. Chrisman SP, Schiff MA, Chung SK, Herring SA, Rivara FP. Implementation of concussion legislation and extent of concussion education for athletes, parents, and coaches in washington state. Am J Sports Med. 2014;42(5):1190–6.
79. Shanley E, Thigpen C, Kissenberth M, Gilliland RG, Thorpe J, Nance D, et al. Heads up football training decreases concussion rates in high school football players. Clin J Sport Med. 2021;31(2):120–6.

Index

.